Minimally Invasive Intracranial Surgery

Guest Editors

MICHAEL E. SUGHRUE, MD
CHARLES TEO, MD

NEUROSURGERY
CLINICS OF NORTH AMERICA

www.neurosurgery.theclinics.com

Consulting Editors
ANDREW T. PARSA, MD, PhD
PAUL C. McCORMICK, MD, MPH

October 2010 • Volume 21 • Number 4

SAUNDERS an imprint of ELSEVIER, Inc.

W.B. SAUNDERS COMPANY
A Division of Elsevier Inc.

1600 John F. Kennedy Blvd. • Suite 1800 • Philadelphia, PA 19103-2899

http://www.theclinics.com

NEUROSURGERY CLINICS OF NORTH AMERICA Volume 21, Number 4
October 2010 ISSN 1042-3680, ISBN-13: 978-1-4377-2469-1

Editor: Ruth Malwitz
Developmental Editor: Donald Mumford

Neurosurgery Clinics of North America (ISSN 1042-3680) is published quarterly by Elsevier Inc., 360 Park Avenue South, New York, NY 10010-1710. Months of issue are January, April, July, and October. Business and Editorial Offices: 1600 John F. Kennedy Blvd., Suite 1800, Philadelphia, PA 19103-2899. Customer Service Office: 11830 Westline Industrial Drive, St. Louis, MO 63146. Periodicals postage paid at New York, NY, and additional mailing offices. Subscription prices are $317.00 per year (US individuals), $492.00 per year (US institutions), $347.00 per year (Canadian individuals), $601.00 per year (Canadian institutions), $443.00 per year (international individuals), $601.00 per year (international institutions), $156.00 per year (US students), and $214.00 per year (international students). International air speed delivery is included in all *Clinics* subscription prices. All prices are subject to change without notice. **POSTMASTER:** Send address changes to *Neurosurgery Clinics of North America*, Elsevier Periodicals Customer Service, 11830 Westline Industrial Drive, St. Louis, MO 63146. **Customer Service: 1-800-654-2452 (US and Canada). From outside the US and Canada, call: 1-314-453-7041. Fax: 1-314-453-5170. E-mail: JournalsCustomerService-usa@elsevier.com (for print support) and journalsonlinesupport-usa@elsevier.com (for online support).**

Reprints. For copies of 100 or more, of articles in this publication, please contact the Commercial Reprints Department, Elsevier Inc., 360 Park Avenue South, New York, NY 10010-1710. Tel. (212) 633-3812; Fax: (212) 462-1935; E-mail: reprints@elsevier.com.

Neurosurgery Clinics of North America is covered in *MEDLINE/PubMed (Index Medicus), EMBASE/Excerpta Medica, and Current Contents/Clinical Medicine (CC/CM).*

Contributors

CONSULTING EDITORS

ANDREW T. PARSA, MD, PhD
Associate Professor; Principal Investigator,
Brain Tumor Research Center; Reza and
Georgianna Khatib Endowed Chair in Skull
Base Tumor Surgery, Department of
Neurological Surgery, University of California,
San Francisco, San Francisco, California

PAUL C. MCCORMICK, MD, MPH, FACS
Herbert & Linda Gallen Professor of
Neurological Surgery, Department of
Neurological Surgery, Columbia University
Medical Center, New York, New York

GUEST EDITORS

MICHAEL E. SUGHRUE, MD
Department of Neurological Surgery,
University of California, San Francisco,
San Francisco, California

CHARLES TEO, MD
Director, Centre for Minimally Invasive
Neurosurgery, POW Private Hospital,
Randwick, New South Wales, Australia

AUTHORS

MANISH K. AGHI, MD, PhD
Department of Neurological Surgery,
University of California, San Francisco,
San Francisco, California

MARVIN BERGSNEIDER, MD
Professor, Department of Neurosurgery,
David Geffen School of Medicine at University
of California, Los Angeles, Los Angeles,
California

RICARDO L. CARRAU, MD
Neuroscience Institute and Brain Tumor
Center, John Wayne Cancer Institute, Saint
John's Health Center, Santa Monica,
California

GIACOMO CONSIGLIERI, MD
Resident, Division of Neurological Surgery,
Barrow Neurological Institute, St Joseph's
Hospital and Medical Center, Phoenix, Arizona

LEO F.S. DITZEL FILHO, MD
Neuroscience Institute and Brain Tumor
Center, John Wayne Cancer Institute, Saint
John's Health Center, Santa Monica, California

LARS FÜLLBIER, MD
Department of Neurosurgery,
Katharinenhospital, Stuttgart, Germany

GARY L. GALLIA, MD, PhD
Assistant Professor of Neurosurgery and
Oncology; Director, Endoscopic and Minimally
Invasive Neurosurgery; Director, Neurosurgery
Skull Base Center, Department of
Neurosurgery, Pituitary Center, Johns Hopkins
Hospital, Baltimore, Maryland

MARK GARRETT, MD
Resident, Division of Neurological Surgery,
Barrow Neurological Institute, St Joseph's
Hospital and Medical Center, Phoenix, Arizona

JEREMY D.W. GREENLEE, MD
Assistant Professor, Department of
Neurosurgery, University of Iowa Hospitals
and Clinics, Iowa City, Iowa

DANIEL J. GUILLAUME, MD, MSc
Assistant Professor, Department of
Neurosurgery, Oregon Health and Science
University, Portland, Oregon

NIKOLAI J. HOPF, MD, PhD
Director, Department of Neurosurgery,
Katharinenhospital, Stuttgart, Germany

MASARU ISHII, MD, PhD
Associate Professor, Department of
Otolaryngology–Head and Neck Surgery,
Johns Hopkins Hospital, Baltimore, Maryland

AMIN B. KASSAM, MD
Neuroscience Institute and Brain Tumor
Center, John Wayne Cancer Institute, Saint
John's Health Center, Santa Monica, California

PAUL S. LARSON, MD
Associate Professor, Department of
Neurological Surgery, University of California,
San Francisco; Chief, Neurosurgery, San
Francisco Veterans Affairs Medical Center, San
Francisco, California

TIMOTHY LINDLEY, MD, PhD
Neurosurgical Resident, Department of
Neurosurgery, University of Iowa Hospitals
and Clinics, Iowa City, Iowa

STEVEN A. MILLS, BFA
Department of Neurological Surgery,
University of California, San Francisco,
San Francisco, California

PETER NAKAJI, MD
Director, Minimally Invasive Neurosurgery;
Director, Neurosurgery Residency Progam,
Division of Neurological Surgery, Barrow
Neurological Institute, St Joseph's Hospital
and Medical Center, Phoenix, Arizona

DANIEL M. PREVEDELLO, MD
Department of Neurological Surgery, The Ohio
State University, Columbus, Ohio

DOMENICO SOLARI, MD
Division of Neurosurgery, Department of
Neurological Sciences, Università degli Studi di
Napoli Federico II, Naples, Italy; Neuroscience
Institute and Brain Tumor Center, John Wayne
Cancer Institute, Saint John's Health Center,
Santa Monica, California

MICHAEL E. SUGHRUE, MD
Department of Neurological Surgery,
University of California, San Francisco,
San Francisco, California

CHARLES TEO, MD
Director, Centre for Minimally Invasive
Neurosurgery, POW Private Hospital,
Randwick, New South Wales, Australia

MARILENE B. WANG, MD
Professor, Division of Head and Neck Surgery,
David Geffen School of Medicine at University
of California, Los Angeles, Los Angeles,
California

ISAAC YANG, MD
Assistant Professor, Department of Surgery,
Harbor-UCLA Medical Center, David Geffen
School of Medicine at University of California,
Los Angeles, Los Angeles, California

RONALD L. YOUNG II, MD
Indianapolis Neurosurgery Group,
Indianapolis, Indiana

Contents

Skull base lesions that involve the middle and posterior cerebral fossae have been historically managed through extensive transcranial approaches. The development of endoscopic endonasal techniques during the past decade has made possible a vast array of alternative routes to the ventral skull base, providing the ability to expose lesions in difficult-to-access regions of the cranial base in a less invasive manner. In this review, the authors detail the endoscopic surgical anatomy and the operative nuances of the expanded endoscopic endonasal approaches to tumors of the middle and posterior cranial fossae. These techniques offer excellent exposure of the targeted regions yielding optimal resections, while avoiding the morbidity associated with transcranial surgical approaches.

Endonasal, endoscopic approaches to the cranial base have undergone significant technique refinement over the past decade. Repair of the resultant defects remains perhaps the most important concern with these approaches; however, recent advances suggest that with careful attention to the closure, these procedures can be done with acceptable rates of morbidity. In this review, the authors discuss known techniques for the repair of endonasal defects, and provide some insight based on their experience.

This article reviews the published experience of others and introduces the authors' insights into the development of an endoscopic pituitary program. While initially challenging, this transition to endoscopic trans-sphenoidal pituitary surgery can yield rewards in the form of superior visualization and potentially more complete tumor resections. With increasing cumulative experience with the endoscopic transsphenoidal technique for pituitary surgery, the improved visualization and less steep learning curve will facilitate more widespread acceptance of endoscopic pituitary surgery as a valid alternative to the trans-septal trans-sphenoidal microscopic approach to pituitary tumors. If not a complete alternative, endoscopic-assisted pituitary surgery will also become more widespread, as endoscopy can easily supplement standard microscopic approaches to pituitary tumors. As transnasal endoscopic approaches to the skull base are increasingly refined in technology and skill, additional applications of this technology may permit skull base approaches through the planum sphenoidale and tuberculum sellae for the removal of giant suprasellar macroadenomas that may otherwise require an open craniotomy for surgical management. The collaboration between otolaryngologists and neurosurgeons is important for further developing successful endoscopic trans-sphenoidal pituitary surgery and improving care for patients. Objective evidence is needed to validate whether the improved visualization results in superior patient outcomes and reduced clinical complications, and if this technique can be reasonably taught in a controlled, supervised setting in residency training programs. Additional outcomes data are needed to evaluate long-term outcomes and define the boundaries of endoscopic trans-sphenoidal pituitary surgery.

This article focuses on minimally invasive approaches used to address disorders of cerebrospinal fluid (CSF) circulation. The author covers the primary CSF disorders that are amenable to minimally invasive treatment, including aqueductal stenosis, fourth ventricular outlet obstruction (including Chiari malformation), isolated lateral ventricle, isolated fourth ventricle, multiloculated hydrocephalus, arachnoid cysts, and tumors that block CSF flow. General approaches to evaluating disorders of CSF circulation, including detailed imaging studies, are discussed. Approaches to minimally invasive management of such disorders are described in general, and for each specific entity. For each procedure, indications, surgical technique, and known outcomes are detailed. Specific complications as well as strategies for their avoidance and management are addressed. Lastly, future directions and the need for structured outcome studies are discussed.

Intracranial vascular lesions are known to affect 2% to 4% of the population, predisposing those affected to a lifetime risk of hemorrhagic stroke, ischemia, focal neurologic deficits, or epileptic seizures. These lesions constitute a heterogeneous group, with different lesion types characterized by distinct biologic mechanisms of pathogenesis and progression. In this article, the minimally invasive management of intracranial aneurysms, arteriovenous malformations including arteriovenous fistulas, and cavernous malformations are discussed.

Movement disorders surgery, particularly deep brain stimulation (DBS), is already a minimally invasive procedure. However, new innovations in the delivery devices for DBS electrodes, new methods for target localization, and alternatives to implanted hardware are all strategies that can make movement disorders surgery less invasive. Frameless DBS techniques can increase patient comfort and shorten operative time. Interventional magnetic resonance imaging can further reduce operative time, and allows DBS placement to be done with a patient asleep and usually with a single brain penetration. Finally, gene transfer eliminates the need for implanted hardware or batteries and simplifies postoperative care.

Although minimally invasive neurosurgery (MIN) holds the potential for reducing the approach-related impact on normal brain, bone, and soft tissues, which must be manipulated in more conventional transcranial microneurosurgery, the techniques necessary to perform minimally invasive, yet maximally effective neurosurgery place significant demands on the surgeon because in many ways the more limited exposure creates a number of unique ways these operations can go wrong. Safe and effective MIN requires the conscious institution of specific alterations to the surgeon's usual operative case flow, which are designed to make specific well-known mistakes impossible or at least very unlikely. Thus, it is important for the aspiring MIN surgeons to learn from the mistakes of their predecessors and to institute patterns of behavior that prevent a repetition of these mistakes. This article provides practical information regarding known pitfalls in intraventricular and transcranial neuroendoscopic surgeries and practical methods to reduce the incidence of these complications to the lowest rate possible.

Neurosurgery Clinics of North America

THE CLINICS ARE NOW AVAILABLE ONLINE!

Access your subscription at:
www.theclinics.com

Neurosurgery Clinics of North America

Preface

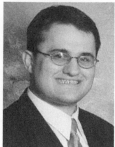
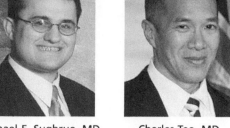

Michael E. Sughrue, MD   Charles Teo, MD
Guest Editors

The present issue of *Neurosurgery Clinics of North America* aims to summarize the rapidly growing range of neurosurgical techniques being utilized worldwide to reduce the impact of intracranial procedures on our patients. Given our belief in the utility of the endoscope in achieving this goal in many situations, many of the articles in this issue focus on endoscopic techniques; however, it is important to point out that not all minimally invasive brain surgeries utilize the endoscope.

However, more importantly, this issue aims to convey a philosophy that is true by definition: namely, that the best surgery for a given lesion is the one that involves the least exposure or manipulation of the brain, neural structures, or critical vessels, yet achieves the goals of surgery. There is widespread consensus in neurosurgery that brain retraction and unnecessary manipulation of the nerves is undesirable, and we believe that the natural extension of these conclusions is that any technique that can achieve the same goal with less brain retraction and neural manipulation is inherently better. What "the least exposure necessary" entails may vary between cases ranging from minimal exposures to more extensive craniotomies; however, the key is that the exposure should be tailored to the needs of the specific patient and be made as minimal as possible.

Being a vocal advocate of minimally invasive intracranial surgery inherently puts one in a position of being an advocate for change, and controversy is an inevitable companion of change. We would propose that given the self-evident advantages of less aggressive surgical approaches, the impressive ability for the nasal cavity to heal, and the potential visualization advantages provided by the endoscope that the arguments should stop being about "traditional" vs "minimally invasive" approaches, or "microscope" vs "endoscope," but instead should be "How do we make minimally invasive surgery work?" It is worth pointing out that the instrumentation, ergonomics, training paradigms, and operative techniques of microneurosurgery are in their mature form, having been refined over the past 50 years. In contrast, many of the approaches and techniques described in this issue are discussed by the surgeons who first pioneered these techniques, highlighting that minimally invasive neurosurgery is a relatively new discipline. The fact that such comparisons are felt worthy of discussion at this early time point along the technologic evolution of minimally invasive surgery, highlights the vast potential these techniques have to improve the care of our patients, and the importance of continued innovation.

Michael E. Sughrue, MD
Department of Neurological Surgery
University of California at San Francisco
505 Parnassus Avenue
San Francisco, CA 94117, USA

Charles Teo, MD
Centre for Minimally Invasive Neurosurgery
POW Private Hospital
Barker Street
Randwick, NSW 2022, Australia

E-mail addresses:
sughruem@neurosurg.ucsf.edu (M.E. Sughrue)
Charlie@neuroendoscopy.info (C. Teo)

Neurosurg Clin N Am 21 (2010) xi
doi:10.1016/j.nec.2010.07.007
1042-3680/10/$ — see front matter © 2010 Elsevier Inc. All rights reserved.

neurosurgery.theclinics.com

The Concept of Minimally Invasive Neurosurgery

Charles Teo, MD

KEYWORDS
- Neurosurgery • Keyhole technique • Minimally invasive
- Neuroendoscopy

All truth passes through 3 stages. First, it is ridiculed; second, it is violently opposed. Third, it is accepted as being self-evident.
                    Schopenhauer (1788–1860)

From the inception of neurosurgery as a separate surgical discipline, there has been a consistent theme in its teachings, that a bigger opening is better. This concept was dogma until only a few decades ago when it was not uncommon to face insurmountable brain swelling on opening the dura. The conditions resulted from a combination of factors, including the use of volatile anesthetic agents, nonselective vasopressors for controlled hypotension, and poor patient positioning as a consequence of cumbersome operative tables and the inability to ideally elevate a patient's head. With this fear of brain swelling came a general philosophy that the cranial opening should be as large as possible to offset the intracranial hypertension. A secondary reason for unnecessarily exposing large areas of brain was the ability to perform partial or complete lobectomies in the case of recalcitrant swelling. Also, without stereotactic guidance, and, in earlier days, without accurate preoperative imaging, it was necessary to expose as much cortical surface as possible in case the surface landmarks were imprecise. Finally, the most commonly cited reason for rejecting smaller craniotomies was the inability to control hemorrhage through a small hole. Collectively, these fears understandably resulted in the teachings of our forefathers. The most commonly performed cranial opening was the frontotemporal craniotomy using a large

question mark incision on the left and a reverse question mark incision on the right. Even other areas of the brain were accessed through large osteoplastic flaps based on the temporalis or the occipitalis muscles. Neurosurgeons in the past did this to expedite the closure in the absence of synthetic bone closing hardware and because a popular dogma at the time was that a vascularized flap was less likely to become infected or necrotic.

In the past 30 years, technological advances have all but eliminated these limitations and fears. Preoperative imaging has become so sophisticated that a surgical approach can be planned with millimeter accuracy, and in some centers on a computerized virtual reality platform. Intraoperative stereotactic guidance may improve that accuracy to the submillimeter and assist with choosing the perfect trajectory to the target lesion. Electric beds with remote controls allow operating room staff to position patients ideally and rapidly even when fully draped. Anesthesiologists are less inclined to use volatile agents and many of the anesthetic drugs used today reduce intracranial pressure rather than increase it. Blood pressure drugs are more selective and less inclined to create cerebral under- or overperfusion. The poor anesthetic conditions once complained of so frequently are a rarity today. Osteoplastic flaps are virtually never performed today because free bone flaps are secured reliably and rapidly with titanium plates. The incidence of infection and bone flap necrosis is low and certainly no higher than that seen with the osteoplastic

Centre for Minimally Invasive Neurosurgery, POW Private Hospital, Barker Street, Randwick, NSW 2022, Australia
E-mail address: Charlie@neuroendoscopy.info

Neurosurg Clin N Am 21 (2010) 583–584
doi:10.1016/j.nec.2010.07.001

flap. Finally, the fear that hemorrhage is less manageable through a small craniotomy than through a large one has been addressed with better bipolar, nonstick forceps and excellent and effective hemostatic agents.

Despite these advances there is still a school of thought that vehemently rejects exposing less brain than is necessary to achieve the goal of surgery. Many of the arguments revolve around statements, such as "I am concerned with damage to the brain, blood vessels and nerves and not the length of the skin incision" or "My results are excellent, why would I change?" or "Cosmetic results and the length of the incision should not take precedence over neurologic outcome". Clearly, the intention of these resistant surgeons is not to insult those surgeons practicing minimally invasive techniques, but the basic premise of their statements implies that surgeons who are minimally invasive are more concerned with cosmetic outcome than neurologic outcome. This is obviously not the case. Indeed, the intention of the minimally invasive neurosurgeon is to improve patient outcomes. Class 1 data that would show a smaller craniotomy is better than a larger craniotomy will never be attained. To ask minimally invasive neurosurgeons to randomize their patients into two groups, one group on whom surgery is performed through an opening as large as is necessary to achieve the intended result as safely and as efficiently as possible and another on whom surgery is performed with the same goals but through an unnecessarily large craniotomy, will never happen. If a surgeon adopts a new approach and a patient has a worse outcome as a direct result of the approach, then clearly he or she needs to re-evaluate the new approach and modify it or revert to the old approach. The eventual approach will be the most minimally invasive operation whether or not it is 3 cm or 6 cm in diameter, through the nose, or through the cranium. If a surgeon has a 100% success rate and a 0% complication rate doing an operation through an eyebrow incision, however, but could do the same operation through the nose with the same results, then why should not that surgeon include the cosmetic outcome in the surgical treatment algorithm?

The aim of this issue is not to convince neurosurgeons that all intracranial pathology can be treated through a cranial opening the size of a coin; it is to demonstrate the techniques that have evolved out of the minimally invasive philosophy. We firmly believe that by minimizing brain exposure and soft tissue manipulation to the absolute minimum needed to achieve the surgical goals, better patient outcomes may be achieved.

Application of Technology for Minimally Invasive Neurosurgery

Masaru Ishii, MD, PhD[a], Gary L. Gallia, MD, PhD[b,c],*

KEYWORDS

- Endoscopy • Minimally invasive neurosurgery
- Neuroendoscopy • Neurosurgery • Skull base
- Technology

The application of endoscopic techniques has changed the field of neurosurgery. The earliest use of an endoscope in neurosurgery dates back 100 years ago when Victor Lespinasse used a cystoscope to fulgurate the choroid plexus in two infants.[1] Twelve years later, Walter Dandy[2] reported the use of a cystoscope to inspect the lateral ventricle and a ventriculoscope to remove and fulgurate the choroid plexus. In 1923, Jason Mixter[3] was the first to report the use of the endoscope to perform a third ventriculostomy. These early neuroendoscopic procedures, however, were limited by poor image quality and suboptimal illumination. With the introduction of microneurosurgical techniques and cerebrospinal fluid shunting procedures, the development and use of the endoscope in neurosurgery decreased.

Numerous technological developments in the 1960s revolutionized endoscopy and formed the basis of current endoscopic systems. The first of these was the invention of a new rod-lens optical system by Harold Hopkins, PhD, in 1959.[4,5] Coupled with the development of the fiberoptic cold-light source by Karl Storz, this led to a new era in endoscopy.[4,5] The development of charge-coupled devices (CCD) was another technological innovation that improved the quality of transmitted images.[6]

In the 1970s, neuroendoscopic procedures were re-examined and reports began surfacing in the neurosurgical literature.[7–11] Over the past few decades, there has been tremendous application of endoscopy to all aspects of neurosurgery.[12–16] Most recently, endoscopic techniques have expanded the armamentarium of skull base neurosurgeons and otolaryngologists in the surgical treatment of skull base pathologies.[17–25] This issue of the *Neurosurgery Clinics of North America* focuses on minimally invasive intracranial neurosurgery. The purpose of this article is to highlight current technologies as well as comment on the transition from microneurosurgical to neuroendoscopic techniques.

ENDOSCOPY IN NEUROSURGERY

Various endoscopic techniques have been described and are generally categorized into endoscopic, endoscopic-assisted, and endoscopic-controlled neurosurgery.[26] In pure endoscopic neurosurgical procedures, instruments are passed through working channels. There are usually

Funding: none.
[a] Department of Otolaryngology, Head and Neck Surgery, Johns Hopkins Hospital, 601 North Caroline Street, Baltimore, MD 21287, USA
[b] Department of Neurosurgery, Johns Hopkins Hospital, 600 North Wolfe Street, Baltimore, MD 21287, USA
[c] Department of Oncology, Johns Hopkins Hospital, 600 North Wolfe Street, Baltimore, MD 21287, USA
* Corresponding author. Department of Neurosurgery, Johns Hopkins Hospital, 600 North Wolfe Street, Baltimore, MD 21287.
E-mail address: ggallia1@jhmi.edu

Neurosurg Clin N Am 21 (2010) 585–594
doi:10.1016/j.nec.2010.07.009
1042-3680/10/$ – see front matter

multiple channels, including one or more for instrumentation and a separate port for irrigation. Endoscopic third ventriculostomy, septum pellucidotomy, cyst/ventricular fenestration, and surgical treatment of intraventricular pathology are examples of pure endoscopic procedures. In endoscopic-assisted neurosurgical procedures, both the microscope and endoscope are used during the same procedure. The endoscope is used for improved visualization or illumination. Instruments are passed along side the endoscope. In endoscopic-controlled neurosurgery, the procedure is performed solely with the endoscope and instruments are passed along side the scope. Endonasal endoscopic skull base surgery is operationally included in this category, though the procedures are performed through the nasal cavity.

There are several types of endoscopes available that are broadly classed as rigid or flexible scopes. Rigid scopes, also referred to as rod lens endoscopes, are more commonly used and are available in a variety of sizes and shaft lengths. Scopes used for transcranial intraventricular procedures are longer than those used for endoscopic-assisted and endoscopic-controlled procedures, and are placed through a sheath that also contains the instrument channel through which the instruments pass (**Fig. 1**). For other endoscopic procedures, the scopes are shorter and are used without the sheath and working ports; instruments are inserted alongside the shaft of the endoscope. The lenses of rigid endoscopes come in various angles of view. The most commonly used endoscope is the 0° scope. Angled scopes of 30°, 45°, and 70° aid in intraoperative visualization (**Fig. 2**).

Flexible endoscopes are also available. Such scopes rely on flexible fiberoptic illumination. These scopes also have operative channels for instrumentation and are used in transcranial endoscopic procedures. One of the main disadvantages of flexible endoscopes is that the quality of the optics is inferior to that of rigid scopes.

In addition to endoscopes, the basic endoscopic set-up also includes a video camera,

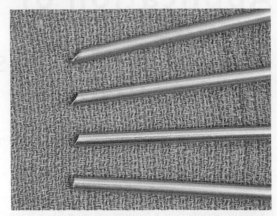

Fig. 2. High-magnification view of the endoscopic lenses, including 0° (*bottom*), 30° (*second from the bottom*), 45°, (*second from the top*), and 70° (*top*).

monitor, light source, and recording devices. The endoscope is connected to the video camera, several of which are available. The majority of current systems use a three-chip CCD. This produces a better quality picture than the single-chip CCD cameras. The picture is then displayed on one or several monitors in the operating room. Recently, high-definition monitors have been introduced that provide spectacular image quality. The current illumination sources used are xenon light sources that are connected to the endoscope via flexible cables. Minimal heat is transmitted through the fiberglass bundles, which significantly reduces thermal injury. Video documentation of intraoperative still photographs or movie clips is extremely valuable, and enables review of operative procedures and serves as a great teaching tool.

A drawback of current monocular endoscopes is that depth perception is impaired when viewing a surgical field.[27] Depth information must be inferred from visual cues and the interaction of surgical instruments with the environment. Stereoscopic endoscopes, endoscopes that can present separate spatially shifted images to the left and right eyes, overcome this limitation by allowing the surgeon to recover natural depth cues from stereo image pairs.[28,29] A number of recent technologic advancements have improved this class of endoscopes and they are now beginning to be used clinically for endoscopic skull base procedures. No differences in surgical time and extent of resection were noted between monocular and stereoscopic matched cases in a recent case series.[29] The inability to rotate an angled scope independently from the image sensor is a limitation of current stereoscopic endoscope designs.

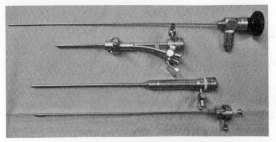

Fig. 1. Rigid 0° endoscope with instrument channel, endoscopic sheath, and associated trocar.

ENDOSCOPIC INSTRUMENTATION

Instruments available for pure endoscopic techniques include scissors, grasping forceps, biopsy forceps, and monopolar and bipolar probes (**Fig. 3**). Additionally, a Fogarty balloon (#3 French) can be passed down in the working channel and is useful for dilation and fenestrations.

Endonasal instruments are varied in number and design (**Fig. 4**), and the instrumentation set may seem overwhelming for staff and novice surgeons at first. There are guidelines, however, that help organize the instruments and simplify instrument choice during surgery. In general, instruments are divided into those that grasp and those that cut. Grasping and cutting instruments are of similar design and structure with the exception of a blade so only cutting instruments are discussed below. Cutting instruments can be further subdivided into scissors and punches. The weight of endoscopic scissors varies; the choice of weight depends on the resilience of the tissue being dissected, with microscissors reserved for cutting

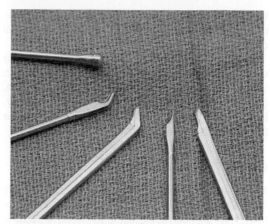

Fig. 4. Endonasal endoscopic instruments, including mushroom punch (*left*), up-biting (*second and third from left*), and straight cutting forceps (*two on right*).

dura and dividing bands during extracapsular dissections, for example. The heaviest scissors are reserved for maneuvers such as turbinate resections. Scissors are curved and straight. We recommend choosing an instrument that places the major axis of the cutting blade perpendicular to the cut direction with the hand placed in the most neutral position.

Punches come in four varieties: straight, up-angled, right-angled, and specialty. Straight instruments place the cutting head in line with the shaft of the instrument. Up-angled deflect the cutting head roughly 45° off line with the shaft of the instrument, while right-angled instruments deflect the biting head 90° off line; that is, they are side-biting. Punches are optimized to cut or divide tissue in plane with the instrument's cutting head, but perform well with any tissue oriented within 45° of the cutting surface. The surgeon must look at a target structure and determine what plane that structure is in with respect to the instrument's shaft and cutting head. The surgeon's goal is to always pick an instrument that places the cutting head inline or parallel with the object she or he is cutting. If, for example, the structure is oriented 45° off axis with the shaft of the instrument then an up-angled instrument is ideal. The degrees of freedom of an instrument in the nose is greatly restricted; that is, one can advance or withdraw an instrument, translate it, or rotate it. It is important to pick the correct instrument because it is hard to compensate for poor instrument choice by instrument manipulation as it is in open surgery.

Specialty instruments have been developed to simplify anterior skull base dissections. These instruments have a bend in the shaft that direct the cutting head toward the skull base. Here the same principles apply orienting the cutting head to

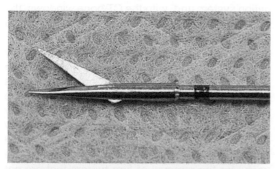

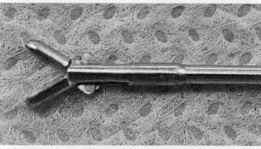

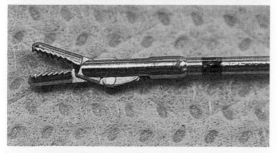

Fig. 3. Endoscopic instruments, including scissors, grasping forceps, and biopsy forceps.

the tissue of interest. Back-biting punches and side-biting punches also exist for addressing special cases.

There are numerous other instruments that have been developed for endonasal skull base surgery. Various blunt and sharp dissectors are available, as well as ring curettes for pituitary tumor surgery. In addition, rotatable microscissors are available for fine sharp dissection.

OTHER TECHNOLOGIES

Microdebriders are commonly used in nasal surgery and represent a major technical advancement for the field. They are used to expeditiously remove tissue in a precise fashion. Originally used by the House group in the 1970s for morselizing acoustic neuromas, microdebriders gained popularity in the orthopedic community for arthroscopic surgery.[30] Setliff[31] and Parsons[32] introduced this technology to nasal surgery in 1994. The basic design of a tissue shaver consists of a hollow shaft attached to a vacuum with a hole at one end. Tissue to be removed is sucked into the hole and sheared off by a rotating, oscillating, or reciprocating inner cannula. The resected tissue and blood are cleared from the surgical field through the hollow shaft. The microdebrider does not alter the morphologic features of the tissue passed though the shaver, making the captured specimens useful for histopathological analysis.[33] Recent advancements in microdebrider technology allow for 360° rotation of the cutting aperture and the ability to control bleeding with bipolar cautery incorporated into the blade. The shaft of the microdebrider blade can either be straight or is available at prebent angles to facilitate access to hard-to-reach areas. Microdebriders have certain limitations that must be recognized. They are inefficient at removing thick bone and, due to their mass and powered nature, they diminish tactile feedback during the removal of soft tissue.[30] Microdebriders are used in the safest fashion when resecting tissue that was deliberately and easily sucked into the cutting aperture. We use them extensively during the approach and often for debulking large tumors. Finer tissue shavers are in development and are better suited for tumor debulking around critical neurovascular structures.

Coblation is an electrosurgical process used to disrupt tissues. There is controversy surrounding the exact mechanism of action of these devices.[34] The major benefit of this technology is its low thermal footprint; that is, it heats the surrounding tissues to a lower temperature[35] (40–70°C) than traditional electrocautery (400°C) devices.[36] This is beneficial when operating near critical structures. Commercial handpieces include a suction port and bipolar cautery. It is hypothesized that the ability to rapidly change between ablation and cautery modes reduce surgery time and blood loss.[36] A recent clinical trial involving skull base and sinonasal tumors supports this conjecture.[37]

Removal of bone is necessary in endoscopic procedures. Pure endoscopic procedures are typically performed via a burr hole. Endoscopic-assisted and transcranial endoscopic-controlled procedures are performed through a craniotomy, often a keyhole craniotomy. The bony work for these procedures is performed with standard perforating drills and craniotomy. For endonasal endoscopic skull base surgery, new drills capable of reaching the skull base have been developed. These drills come in both straight and angled tips. Various burrs are also available, including cutting, diamond, and hybrid bits. For bone removal at the skull base, the hybrid bit is optimal. Recently, irrigation adapters have been developed that help disperse heat when drilling about the optic nerve or other neurovascular structures. The drills can also be registered to the neuronavigation system and, with the CT bone windows, the location along the skull base can be monitored during the bone removal.

Ultrasonic surgical devices were originally developed by the dental industry to remove plaque from hard surfaces.[38,39] In 1967, ophthalmologists started using ultrasonic aspirators to emulsify the lens during cataract surgery.[40,41] Approximately a decade later the technology was adapted by neurosurgeons[42] for the removal of intra-axial and extra-axial tumors. Ultrasonic aspirators are useful for the removal of firm tumors that are not freely suctionable. These devices were modified to disrupt and cut bone[37,39,43–49] and were miniaturized so that they can be used endonasally.[44,45,49] Bone emulsifying aspirators work by delivering vibrations of sufficient amplitude and frequency to disrupt rigid structures. They are designed to exploit differences in tissue properties to minimize injury to soft tissue during the bone emulsification process. This safety feature is not absolute and appropriate technique is required to prevent tissue injury near vital structures.[45,46,50] In general, ultrasonic surgical devices are less efficient at removing bone than drills, so the technology is thought to be complementary rather than a replacement for the drill.[45]

IMAGING: PREOPERATIVE AND INTRAOPERATIVE STEREOTAXIC NEURONAVIGATION

Imaging is essential in all aspect of neurosurgery. Preoperative radiographic evaluations include CT scans, MRI, and angiography. The CT scan is used to define bony anatomy during the approach and the MRI scan is used to provide soft tissue contrast during the tumor resection. Additionally, CT and MRI angiography are useful evaluations. These studies provide information of anatomic landmarks and extent of pathology. Careful review of these studies is crucial for preoperative surgical planning and anticipated intraoperative findings.

Endoscopic surgical landmarks important for identifying vital structures are often distorted or obscured by large skull base lesions. This makes it easy for a surgeon to become disoriented. Disorientation can often be minimized with a systematic surgical approach relying on the sequential identification of important landmarks to maintain orientation. A strong understanding of the three-dimensional surgical anatomy is required to perform these surgeries well. Image-guided surgery is useful in this regard, as it can instantly recall multiplanar reconstructions of a patient's anatomy using images uploaded before

surgery (**Fig. 5**). Often this includes a preoperative MRI scan and CT scan. The disadvantage of this technology is that the preoperative scans lose relevance as the surgery progresses as the surgical process itself changes the anatomy. Intraoperative imaging mitigates this problem (**Fig. 6**). It is thought that intraoperative imaging technologies may enhance the effectiveness of endoscopic procedures and reduce morbidity.[51,52] There are two competing intraoperative imaging modalities: MRI[53–56] and CT scans.[51] In pituitary surgery, intraoperative MRI was shown to identify residual tumor after the surgeon thought tumor resection was complete in 58% to 83% of cases.[54,57,58] The use of intraoperative MRI increased the operative times by 1.8 hours on average. CT scan imaging modalities can be further subdivided into cone beam, multidetector, and fluoroscopy.[52] In general, cone bean CT scanners are smaller, more portable and cheaper than multidetector CT scans. In a similar fashion to intraoperative MRI, intraoperative CT scan was shown to change

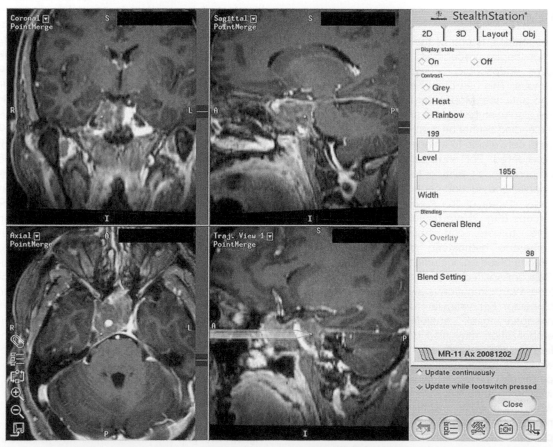

Fig. 5. Intraoperative neuronavigation screenshot during resection of a large pituitary adenoma; taken during the resection of the tumor posterior and lateral to the carotid artery.

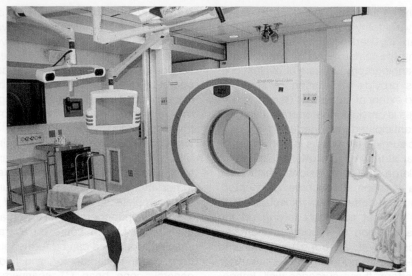

Fig. 6. Intraoperative CT scanner and integrated neuronavigation system.

surgical planning in 24% of endoscopic sinonasal and skull base procedures.[51]

HEMOSTASIS

Hemostasis is one of the major concerns during endoscopic procedures. Most bleeding during pure endoscopic neurosurgical procedures is venous. This can often be managed by irrigation and patience. Monopolar and bipolar coagulation are also useful when the site of bleeding is visible. If bleeding cannot be controlled with these maneuvers, conversion to an open craniotomy should be considered. For endonasal endoscopic surgical procedures, a variety of tools are available.[59] Monopolar and suction cautery are useful during the nasal stages of the surgery. Pistol grip bipolar forceps (**Fig. 7**) are useful for coagulation of the dura, tumors, and small vessels. There are numerous hemostatic materials available for venous bleeding, including microfibrillar collagen, Gelfoam-soaked in thrombin, and oxidized cellulose. Warm irrigation is also effective for mucosal bleeding. For vascular tumors such as juvenile nasopharyngeal angiofibromas, preoperative embolization may also be considered. Injury to large arterial vessels is a major concern especially when the tumor involves these structures. Intraoperatively, the vessel injury site is focally packed with hemostatic materials when possible; in cases where control is unachievable, the vessel may need to be occluded with an aneurysm clip. Any patient with an arterial injury should have a postoperative angiogram and potential definitive endovascular intervention.

FLUORESCEIN

Leakage of cerebrospinal fluid (CSF) into the nasal cavity can lead to life-threatening complications; therefore, it is important to accurately diagnose the presence of a CSF fistula. Several clinical tests can be used to confirm the diagnoses and generally fall into two categories: biochemical analysis (beta 2 transferrin and beta trace) and radiographic methods (CT scan imaging, MRI, and nuclear medicine imaging). Often a combination of techniques is used. Once the diagnosis is confirmed, the precise location of the leak must be identified for repair. Introduced by Kirchner and Proud[60] in 1960, intrathecal fluorescein injection is a commonly used method for localizing low-flow and intermittent leaks. Sodium fluorescein is a fluorescent compound[61] that dyes the CSF green so

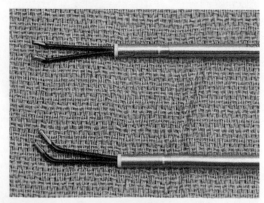

Fig. 7. Pistol grip endoscopic bipolar forceps come in various tip configurations and are essential for precise coagulation.

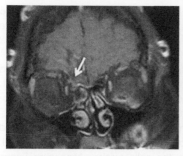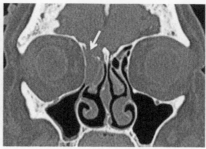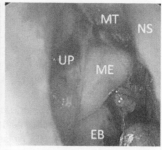

Fig. 8. From left to right, a coronal T1-weighted MRI scan, a coronal CT scan, and an endoscopic intraoperative image taken with a zero-degree endoscope. The CT scan and MRI scan correspond roughly to the same coronal slice. The images show a skull base defect (*arrows*) and a meningoencephalocele (ME). The endoscopic images show the ME turning green as it fills with fluorescein. EB, ethmoid bulla; MT, middle turbinate; NS, nasal septum; UP, uncinate process.

that it is easier to visualize as it leaks into the nose (**Fig. 8**). Fluorescein injection has not been approved by the US Food and Drug Administration for intrathecal injection and one must be aware of the complications associated with its use and appropriately inform patients of rare, but serious, side effects.[62–68] Paraparesis, numbness, and seizure are the most commonly reported side effects.[69] These are attributed to the injection of too much or too high a concentration of fluorescein,[70] the injection of fluorescein too rapidly, and the use of unsuitable fluorescein preparations.[70] Myelopathy with paraplegia has been reported.[69] Some investigators advocate the use of topical fluorescein as a method for reducing the side-effect profile of the intrathecal approach.[71]

CONVERSION FROM MICROSCOPIC TO ENDOSCOPIC PROCEDURES

As described in other articles in this issue, the endoscope has become an essential tool for neurosurgeons and there has been tremendous applications in the field of neurosurgery. As with any new surgical advancement, there is a learning curve in minimally invasive and endoscopic techniques to become proficient. This learning curve is steep for endoscopic procedures for many reasons. Endoscopic procedures are performed in three-dimensional space but viewed on two-dimensional monitors. As such, depth perception is challenging for the beginner. For endoscopic procedures, new and often unfamiliar instrumentation is required and operative times are significantly longer during the initial endoscopic cases. Additionally, for endonasal skull base procedures, the anatomy is initially unfamiliar.

As minimally invasive centers continue to grow, future generations of neurosurgeons and otolaryngologists will be trained in and become proficient

with endoscopic procedures. For surgeons who are interested in mastering such techniques, some recommendations are suggested. Dedicated anatomic dissections and minimally invasive and endoscopic cadaveric courses are crucial to become more familiar with the surgical anatomy and the instrumentation. A good initial strategy is to gradually increase endoscopic use with each successive case until the entire procedure is performed endoscopically. Additionally, it is important to identify cases appropriate to the level of surgical skill. This has been nicely described by the Pittsburgh group, which has developed a training plan for acquisition of endonasal endoscopic surgical skill. This consists of a modular and incremental approach based on the difficulty of the procedure in which surgeons should not progress to the next level unless the current level of cases has been mastered.[72]

SUMMARY

The development of modern endoscopy has impacted every aspect of neurosurgery. This article highlights current technological developments, including endoscopic instrumentation and devices, imaging, and hemostatic agents. Future technologies, including robotic surgery, virtual endoscopy, and surgical simulation, will further expand the possibilities and applications of endoscopy in our field.

REFERENCES

1. Grant JA. Victor Darwin Lespinasse: a biographical sketch. Neurosurgery 1996;39(6):1232–3.
2. Dandy W. Cerebral ventriculoscopy. Bull Johns Hopkins Hosp 1922;38:189.
3. Mixter W. Ventriculoscopy and puncture of the floor of the third ventricle. Boston Med Surg J 1923;188: 277–8.

4. Cockett WS, Cockett AT. The Hopkins rod-lens system and the Storz cold light illumination system. Urology 1998;51(Suppl 5A):1–2.

5. Linder TE, Simmen D, Stool SE. Revolutionary inventions in the 20th century. The history of endoscopy. Arch Otolaryngol Head Neck Surg 1997;123(11):1161–3.

6. Boyle W, Smith GE. Charge couple semiconductor devices. Bell System Tech J 1970;49:587–93.

7. Apuzzo ML, Heifetz MD, Weiss MH, et al. Neurosurgical endoscopy using the side-viewing telescope. J Neurosurg 1977;46(3):398–400.

8. Fukushima T. Endoscopic biopsy of intraventricular tumors with the use of a ventriculofiberscope. Neurosurgery 1978;2(2):110–3.

9. Fukushima T, Ishijima B, Hirakawa K, et al. Ventriculofiberscope: a new technique for endoscopic diagnosis and operation. Technical note. J Neurosurg 1973;38(2):251–6.

10. Vries JK. An endoscopic technique for third ventriculostomy. Surg Neurol 1978;9(3):165–8.

11. Vries JK. Endoscopy as an adjunct to shunting for hydrocephalus. Surg Neurol 1980;13(1):69–72.

12. Cappabianca P, Cinalli G, Gangemi M, et al. Application of neuroendoscopy to intraventricular lesions. Neurosurgery 2008;62(Suppl 2):575–97 [discussion: 597–8].

13. Fries G, Perneczky A. Endoscope-assisted brain surgery: part 2—analysis of 380 procedures. Neurosurgery 1998;42(2):226–31 [discussion: 231–2].

14. Perneczky A, Boecher-Schwarz HG. Endoscope-assisted microsurgery for cerebral aneurysms. Neurol Med Chir (Tokyo) 1998;38(Suppl):33–4.

15. Perneczky A, Fries G. Endoscope-assisted brain surgery: part 1—evolution, basic concept, and current technique. Neurosurgery 1998;42(2):219–24 [discussion: 224–5].

16. Cinalli G, Cappabianca P, de Falco R, et al. Current state and future development of intracranial neuroendoscopic surgery. Expert Rev Med Devices 2005;2(3):351–73.

17. Cappabianca P, Cavallo LM, Esposito F, et al. Extended endoscopic endonasal approach to the midline skull base: the evolving role of transsphenoidal surgery. Adv Tech Stand Neurosurg 2008;33:151–99.

18. Kassam A, Thomas AJ, Snyderman C, et al. Fully endoscopic expanded endonasal approach treating skull base lesions in pediatric patients. J Neurosurg 2007;106(Suppl 2):75–86.

19. Snyderman CH, Carrau RL, Kassam AB, et al. Endoscopic skull base surgery: principles of endonasal oncological surgery. J Surg Oncol 2008;97(8):658–64.

20. Snyderman CH, Pant H, Carrau RL, et al. What are the limits of endoscopic sinus surgery?: the expanded endonasal approach to the skull base. Keio J Med 2009;58(3):152–60.

21. Schwartz TH, Fraser JF, Brown S, et al. Endoscopic cranial base surgery: classification of operative approaches. Neurosurgery 2008;62(5):991–1002 [discussion: 1002–5].

22. Kassam A, Snyderman CH, Mintz A, et al. Expanded endonasal approach: the rostrocaudal axis. Part II. Posterior clinoids to the foramen magnum. Neurosurg Focus 2005;19(1):E4.

23. Kassam A, Snyderman CH, Mintz A, et al. Expanded endonasal approach: the rostrocaudal axis. Part I. Crista galli to the sella turcica. Neurosurg Focus 2005;19(1):E3.

24. Cavallo LM, Messina A, Cappabianca P, et al. Endoscopic endonasal surgery of the midline skull base: anatomical study and clinical considerations. Neurosurg Focus 2005;19(1):E2.

25. Cavallo LM, Messina A, Gardner P, et al. Extended endoscopic endonasal approach to the pterygopalatine fossa: anatomical study and clinical considerations. Neurosurg Focus 2005;19(1):E5.

26. Hopf NJ, Perneczky A. Endoscopic neurosurgery and endoscope-assisted microneurosurgery for the treatment of intracranial cysts. Neurosurgery 1998;43(6):1330–6 [discussion: 1336–7].

27. Chan AC, Chung SC, Yim AP, et al. Comparison of two-dimensional vs three-dimensional camera systems in laparoscopic surgery. Surg Endosc 1997;11(5):438–40.

28. Fraser JF, Allen B, Anand VK, et al. Three-dimensional neurostereoendoscopy: subjective and objective comparison to 2D. Minim Invasive Neurosurg 2009;52(1):25–31.

29. Tabaee A, Anand VK, Fraser JF, et al. Three-dimensional endoscopic pituitary surgery. Neurosurgery 2009;64(5 Suppl 2):288–93 [discussion: 294–5].

30. Bruggers S, Sindwani R. Innovations in microdebrider technology and design. Otolaryngol Clin North Am 2009;42(5):781–7, viii.

31. Setliff RC 3rd. The hummer: a remedy for apprehension in functional endoscopic sinus surgery. Otolaryngol Clin North Am 1996;29(1):95–104.

32. Parsons DS. Rhinologic uses of powered instrumentation in children beyond sinus surgery. Otolaryngol Clin North Am 1996;29(1):105–14.

33. Zweig JL, Schaitkin BM, Fan CY, et al. Histopathology of tissue samples removed using the microdebrider technique: implications for endoscopic sinus surgery. Am J Rhinol 2000;14(1):27–32.

34. Zinder DJ. Common myths about electrosurgery. Otolaryngol Head Neck Surg 2000;123(4):450–5.

35. Palmer JM. Bipolar radiofrequency for adenoidectomy. Otolaryngol Head Neck Surg 2006;135(2):323–4.

36. Swibel Rosenthal LH, Benninger MS, Stone CH, et al. Wound healing in the rabbit paranasal sinuses after Coblation: evaluation for use in endoscopic

sinus surgery. Am J Rhinol Allergy 2009;23(3): 360–3.

37. Kostrzewa JP, Sunde J, Riley KO, et al. Radiofre-quency coblation decreases blood loss during endoscopic sinonasal and skull base tumor removal. ORL J Otorhinolaryngol Relat Spec 2010;72(1): 38–43.

38. Jallo GI. CUSA EXcel ultrasonic aspiration system. Neurosurgery 2001;48(3):695–7.

39. Kim K, Isu T, Morimoto D, et al. Anterior vertebral artery decompression with an ultrasonic bone curette to treat bow hunter's syndrome. Acta Neuro-chir (Wien) 2008;150(3):301–3 [discussion: 303].

40. Kelman CD. Phaco-emulsification and aspiration. A new technique of cataract removal. A preliminary report. Am J Ophthalmol 1967;64(1):23–35.

41. Kelman CD. Phaco-emulsification and aspiration. A progress report. Am J Ophthalmol 1969;67(4): 464–77.

42. Flamm ES, Ransohoff J, Wuchinich D, et al. Prelimi-nary experience with ultrasonic aspiration in neuro-surgery. Neurosurgery 1978;2(3):240–5.

43. Abe T. New devices for direct transnasal surgery on pituitary adenomas. Biomed Pharmacother 2002;56(Suppl 1):171s–7s.

44. Bolger WE. Piezoelectric surgical device in endo-scopic sinus surgery: an initial clinical experience. Ann Otol Rhinol Laryngol 2009;118(9):621–4.

45. Cappabianca P, Cavallo LM, Esposito I, et al. Bone removal with a new ultrasonic bone curette during endoscopic endonasal approach to the sellar-suprasellar area: technical note. Neurosurgery 2010;66(3 Suppl Operative):E118 [discussion: E118].

46. Ito K, Ishizaka S, Sasaki T, et al. Safe and minimally invasive laminoplastic laminotomy using an ultra-sonic bone curette for spinal surgery: technical note. Surg Neurol 2009;72(5):470–5 [discussion: 475].

47. Pagella F, Giourgos G, Matti E, et al. Removal of a fronto-ethmoidal osteoma using the sonopet omni ultrasonic bone curette: first impressions. Laryngoscope 2008;118(2):307–9.

48. Samy RN, Krishnamoorthy K, Pensak ML. Use of a novel ultrasonic surgical system for decompres-sion of the facial nerve. Laryngoscope 2007; 117(5):872–5.

49. Yamasaki T, Moritake K, Nagai H, et al. A new, mini-ature ultrasonic surgical aspirator with a handpiece designed for transsphenoidal surgery. Technical note. J Neurosurg 2003;99(1):177–9.

50. Chang HS, Joko M, Song JS, et al. Ultrasonic bone curettage for optic canal unroofing and anterior cli-noidectomy. Technical note. J Neurosurg 2006; 104(4):621–4.

51. Batra PS, Kanowitz SJ, Citardi MJ. Clinical utility of intraoperative volume computed tomography

scanner for endoscopic sinonasal and skull base procedures. Am J Rhinol 2008;22(5):511–5.

52. Isaacs S, Fakhri S, Luong A, et al. Intraoperative imaging for otorhinolaryngology-head and neck surgery. Otolaryngol Clin North Am 2009;42(5): 765–79, viii.

53. Baumann F, Schmid C, Bernays RL. Intraoperative magnetic resonance imaging-guided transsphenoi-dal surgery for giant pituitary adenomas. Neurosurg Rev 2010;33(1):83–90.

54. Wu JS, Shou XF, Yao CJ, et al. Transsphenoidal pitu-itary macroadenomas resection guided by PoleStar N20 low-field intraoperative magnetic resonance imaging: comparison with early postoperative high-field magnetic resonance imaging. Neurosurgery 2009;65(1):63–70 [discussion: 70–1].

55. Ntoukas V, Krishnan R, Seifert V. The new generation polestar n20 for conventional neurosurgical oper-ating rooms: a preliminary report. Neurosurgery 2008;62(3 Suppl 1):82–9 [discussion: 89–90].

56. Sutherland GR, Kaibara T, Louw D, et al. A mobile high-field magnetic resonance system for neurosur-gery. J Neurosurg 1999;91(5):804–13.

57. Gerlach R, du Mesnil de Rochemont R, Gasser T, et al. Feasibility of Polestar N20, an ultra-low-field intraoperative magnetic resonance imaging system in resection control of pituitary macroadenomas: lessons learned from the first 40 cases. Neurosur-gery 2008;63(2):272–84 [discussion: 284–5].

58. Lewin JS, Nour SG, Meyers ML, et al. Intraoperative MRI with a rotating, tiltable surgical table: a time use study and clinical results in 122 patients. AJR Am J Roentgenol 2007;189(5):1096–103.

59. Kassam A, Snyderman CH, Carrau RL, et al. En-doneurosurgical hemostasis techniques: lessons learned from 400 cases. Neurosurg Focus 2005; 19(1):E7.

60. Kirchner FR, Proud GO. Method for the identification and localization of cerebrospinal fluid, rhinorrhea and otorrhea. Laryngoscope 1960;70:921–31.

61. Felisati G, Bianchi A, Lozza P, et al. Italian multi-centre study on intrathecal fluorescein for cranio-sinusal fistulae. Acta Otorhinolaryngol Ital 2008; 28(4):159–63.

62. Anari S, Waldron M, Carrie S. Delayed absence seizure: a complication of intrathecal fluorescein injection. A case report and literature review. Auris Nasus Larynx 2007;34(4):515–8.

63. Coeytaux A, Reverdin A, Jallon P, et al. Non convul-sive status epilepticus following intrathecal fluores-cein injection. Acta Neurol Scand 1999;100(4): 278–80.

64. Keerl R, Weber RK, Draf W, et al. Use of sodium fluo-rescein solution for detection of cerebrospinal fluid fistulas: an analysis of 420 administrations and re-ported complications in Europe and the United States. Laryngoscope 2004;114(2):266–72.

65. Locatelli D, Rampa F, Acchiardi I, et al. Endoscopic endonasal approaches for repair of cerebrospinal fluid leaks: nine-year experience. Neurosurgery 2006;58(4 Suppl 2):ONS246–56 [discussion: ONS-256–7].

66. Moseley JI, Carton CA, Stern WE. Spectrum of complications in the use of intrathecal fluorescein. J Neurosurg 1978;48(5):765–7.

67. Placantonakis DG, Tabaee A, Anand VK, et al. Safety of low-dose intrathecal fluorescein in endoscopic cranial base surgery. Neurosurgery 2007;61(Suppl 3):161–5 [discussion: 165–6].

68. Wallace JD, Weintraub MI, Mattson RH, et al. Status epilepticus as a complication of intrathecal fluorescein. Case report. J Neurosurg 1972;36(5): 659–60.

69. Park KY, Kim YB. A case of myelopathy after intrathecal injection of fluorescein. J Korean Neurosurg Soc 2007;42(6):492–4.

70. Wolf G, Greistorfer K, Stammberger H. [Endoscopic detection of cerebrospinal fluid fistulas with a fluorescence technique. Report of experiences with over 925 cases]. Laryngorhinootologie 1997;76(10): 588–94 [in German].

71. Saafan ME, Ragab SM, Albirmawy OA. Topical intranasal fluorescein: the missing partner in algorithms of cerebrospinal fluid fistula detection. Laryngoscope 2006;116(7):1158–61.

72. Snyderman C, Kassam A, Carrau R, et al. Acquisition of surgical skills for endonasal skull base surgery: a training program. Laryngoscope 2007; 117(4):699–705.

Transcranial Minimally Invasive Neurosurgery for Tumors

Mark Garrett, MD, Giacomo Consiglieri, MD,
Peter Nakaji, MD*

KEYWORDS

- Neuroendoscopy • Neurosurgery • Transcranial
- Minimally invasive

The concept of a "minimally invasive approach," when applied to neuro-oncological surgery, continues to excite controversy. The debate over what type of approach should be used often hinges on whether a small craniotomy is intrinsically less invasive or whether a larger craniotomy results in less morbidity and therefore is a more appropriate choice. The most common goals of neuro-oncological surgery are to obtain a diagnosis, to achieve maximum tumor reduction, and to avoid neurologic deficits. Whether these goals can be accomplished as well as or better through minimally invasive approaches often cannot be answered meaningfully without large and well-designed clinical studies, which are as lacking in this field as in many other fields of neurosurgery. A similar problem exists for the related field of endoscopic intracranial extraventricular surgery in general.

The avid practitioner of minimally invasive and endoscopic neurosurgery often wryly considers the history of microneurosurgery, in which pioneer users of the operating microscope, such as Kurze, Pool, and Yasargil, had to convince skeptical colleagues of the value of microscopy, which is now accepted as a standard of care in many cases. Adherents to the minimally invasive philosophy believe that excellent outcomes can be achieved by coupling keyhole approaches and the endoscope in cases traditionally approached through larger craniotomies. In this age, the idea of a tailored craniotomy that exactly fits the pathologic condition, rather than a standard or one-size-fits-all approach, should not seem revolutionary. As for the endoscope, it is simply a tool for enhancing visualization. Neurosurgeons should welcome any tool that improves visualization.

This article discusses common minimally invasive craniotomy approaches and the role of neuroendoscopy in the removal of extra-axial and intra-axial brain tumors, excluding those of the ventricle. The use of the transsphenoidal and extended transsphenoidal approaches is considered only briefly, because they are addressed elsewhere in this issue.

HISTORY

Minimally invasive cranial neurosurgery represents a history of challenges and periodic successes. For decades, the primary concern of neurosurgery has been to minimize the neurovascular impact of surgery. Adequate exposures, which have usually

Division of Neurological Surgery, Barrow Neurological Institute, St Joseph's Hospital and Medical Center, 350 West Thomas Road, Phoenix, AZ 85013, USA
* Corresponding author. c/o Neuroscience Publications, Barrow Neurological Institute, 350 West Thomas Road, Phoenix, AZ 85013.
E-mail address: neuropub@chw.edu

Neurosurg Clin N Am 21 (2010) 595–605
doi:10.1016/j.nec.2010.07.002

meant large exposures, were seen as the key to good outcomes. Skull base microsurgery developed around the belief that better outcomes are achieved by moving bone and soft tissue rather than brain and nerves. The minimally invasive neurosurgery paradigm evolved out of the recognition by many surgeons that, in many cases, they did not use or need much of the exposure provided by extensive approaches, and they began to seek alternatives to the soft tissue trauma, healing, and recovery time involved with extensive approaches. To this end, a few pioneers began to explore smaller approaches to achieve the same neurosurgical goals.

One such approach, the supraorbital transbrow craniotomy, was an adaptation of the orbitozygomatic approach first proposed by Jane and colleagues.[1,2] Popularized by Reisch and Perneczky[4] and by Jho,[3] the technique has become widely practiced by some schools of neurosurgery but has not been accepted universally. The minimally invasive keyhole principles promulgated by these practitioners have gradually been applied to other areas of cranial neurosurgery, where they excite ongoing debate.

Neuroendoscopy has been the foundation of many minimally invasive approaches, although it too has had an on-again, off-again history. In neurosurgical terms, most of the applications of neuroendoscopy proposed to date have been focused on addressing intraventricular pathologies.[5] The first description of a neuroendoscopy procedure was by L'Espinasse in 1910. As described by Walker,[6] L'Espinasse cauterized the choroid plexus in 2 hydrocephalic infants with the assistance of a cystoscope. Dandy[7] described his use of the endoscope to remove the choroid plexus, with results that were similar to those of his experience with formal craniotomy for open choroid plexectomy. The growth of neuroendoscopy was slowed by the significant limitations associated with the lighting and magnification available for early endoscopes. Furthermore, the advent of ventricular shunts and advances in microneurosurgery reduced interest in neuroendoscopy.

In the 1960s and 1970s, technological advances in lens development and the application of fiberoptics improved neuroendoscopic visualization significantly. In 1963, Guiot and colleagues[8] used ventriculoscopy to explore a patient with a colloid cyst. In 1973, Fukushima and colleagues[9] described the first ventricular biopsy. In 1983, Powell and colleagues[10] reported the first endoscopic resection of a colloid cyst, and the technique was popularized throughout the late 1990s.[11–13] The use of endoscopy to address selected intraventricular tumors for biopsy or resection is now a widely accepted therapeutic option.[5]

Subsequently, the application of minimally invasive principles and endoscopy to extra-axial tumors was popularized by Perneczky and Fries.[14] They promoted the endoscope as a means to minimize retraction on the brain and to avoid resection of the dura and bone, which they argued increased operative time and operation-related trauma. In 1998, Fries and Perneczky[15] reported 380 endoscope-assisted cases, 242 of which involved either the subarachnoid space or the cerebral parenchyma. The investigators found that endoscopy improved visualization of perforators during aneurysm surgery and permitted exploration of the ventral brainstem, ventral side of cranial nerves, and ventral aspect of the cervical spine while minimizing retraction. They reported no complications associated with the use of the endoscope itself.

Endoscopic transsphenoidal surgery has been the largest area of recent growth in neuroendoscopy. The field was pioneered by Guiot and colleagues,[8] although Guiot later abandoned it because visualization was poor. In the 1970s the use of neuroendoscopy was again reported[16,17] as an adjuvant to transsphenoidal microneurosurgery, but it was not until 1992 that Jankowski and colleagues[18] reported a purely endoscopic transsphenoidal approach to the sella turcica. Jho and Carrau,[19] who are considered early pioneers of the field, reported 46 purely endoscopic endonasal procedures in 1997. This area continues to expand rapidly, with an increasing number of intradural lesions being approached through an endonasal route. This topic is explored more fully elsewhere in this issue.

The most recent intracranial application of neuroendoscopy is endoscopic resection of intraparenchymal brain tumors. In 2008, Greenfield and colleagues[20] described the use of METRx tubular retractors (Medtronic Inc, Memphis, TN, USA) in combination with frameless stereotactic navigation for complication-free removal of 10 deep lesions. The next year, Kassam and colleagues[21] reported the use of a nonfixed transparent conduit to remove 21 subcortical lesions with no new neurologic complications.

The forays from the ventricles into the subarachnoid and intraparenchymal spaces hardly constitute a mature field. However, these forays are an intriguing direction for minimally invasive neurosurgery. The remainder of this article considers the current state of and future applications for minimally invasive and neuroendoscopic neurosurgery beyond the intraventricular and endonasal routes.

INDICATIONS

The general indications for a minimally invasive approach are the same as those for any other neurosurgical approach to a given tumor. Often the decision to use a keyhole approach depends more on the specific pathologic condition and on the practitioner's experience than on any other factor. Although use of the endoscope depends entirely on the specifics of a case, the addition of the endoscope is often complementary in many keyhole approaches.

The appropriate trajectory is the single most important factor in the success of a minimally invasive tumor approach. Various factors must be considered: (1) the planned extent of resection for the tumor being addressed (complete removal vs debulking vs biopsy); (2) the nature of the tumor involved, particularly the distinction between the tumor and normal brain tissue; (3) the vascularity of the tumor and whether vascular control can be achieved from the chosen trajectory; (4) the surface structures that will be penetrated and whether cosmesis or intervening structures (eg, venous sinuses or bony sinuses) may force deviation from an otherwise ideal trajectory; and (5) the depth of the tumor, which at times can prevent the lesion from being accessed via a small craniotomy. The 2-point method is a simple technique for estimating the best trajectory.[22] A point is placed at the geographic center of the lesion, and a second point is placed where the lesion comes closest to the surface. A line drawn through these 2 points to the surface of the head constitutes the best approach trajectory, subject to modification by the previously mentioned considerations.

The absolute minimum size of the craniotomy is constrained by the instruments that will be used, but it typically is no smaller than the size of an open bipolar forceps.

NEUROENDOSCOPY: APPROACH OR ADJUNCT?

The decision to apply neuroendoscopy to a given tumor surgery requires a major distinction to be made, that is, whether the operation is endoscopically controlled, whereby the endoscope is the sole or primary means of visualization, or whether it is endoscopically assisted. In the latter, microsurgical techniques are the mainstay of dissection and tumor resection, while endoscopy is used to help visualize areas of the tumor that are otherwise difficult to see with the uniaxial view provided by the operative microscope. Endoscopy is also used to examine the tumor bed for completeness

of resection. With image injection, endoscopic images can be inserted into the microscope eyepiece, allowing both to be used together. Many surgeons, however, find this technique to be distracting.[23]

Endoscopically controlled techniques have become the approach of choice for many neurosurgeons for transsphenoidal surgery.[24–28] In most of these applications, the microscope is never used during the operation. A completely endoscopic surgical approach is less commonly used during transcranial neurosurgery. The nose is lined with mucosa, and the risk of damaging structures as one passes instruments is low. Two surgeons can work in concert, introducing and removing instruments with ease. In the cranium, the corridor to the tumor is often lined with brain and neurovascular structures, which poorly tolerate even slight manipulation by passing endoscopes or instruments. Furthermore, the microscope provides an excellent view in a direct line and frees both hands to participate in the dissection. In contrast, in these applications the endoscope often occupies the space of 1 instrument and must be held by the primary surgeon. Therefore, the endoscope tends to be used in a supporting role after access is obtained through microneurosurgery.

However, with a holder or a good assistant, 2-handed work is possible through the endoscope. The instruments are introduced along the endoscope and kept just in front of its tip so that they are always in view. This technique differs from the purely endoscopic approach, in which the instruments travel through the shaft of the endoscope, as is common in intraventricular endoscopic surgery. In the endoscopically assisted technique, the endoscope can be used in multiple stages to inspect the approach, better define the anatomy, see parts of the tumor not in the direct line of vision, and inspect the tumor bed for residual tumor. Particularly, when combined with minimally invasive approaches, smaller craniotomies, and an effort to preserve overlying neural structures, the advantage of the endoscope for working in small spaces and for seeing angles perpendicular to the line of sight can be invaluable. In some instances, both intracranial extra-axial and intra-axial tumors have been removed without the use of the microscope in an endoscopically controlled fashion, but doing so remains relatively unusual.

During tumor resection, the endoscope may be valuable for removing a small amount of residual tumor in a difficult location. For example, Chang and colleagues[29] reported the use of the endoscope to remove the last fragments of a large ecchordosis physaliphora from the clivus that could not be seen with the microscope.

EQUIPMENT

For endoscopically assisted or endoscopically controlled tumor surgery, handheld endoscopes are used and usually held in the nondominant hand or in a rigid holder. Various endoscopes are available. In the authors' opinion, the most suitable endoscope for endoscopically assisted intracranial surgery is the Perneczky endoscope. The right-angle pistol-grip configuration of this endoscope allows it to be held comfortably in the hand for long periods. The rigid shaft of the endoscope allows precise control of its position.

The endoscope is usually held in one hand while the other hand is used for working. An assistant can also hold the endoscope, freeing the surgeon to work with both hands. If needed, the endoscope can be fixated with the use of one of many available retractor arms (see another article elsewhere in this issue). Many other types of endoscopes can be used for endoscopically assisted or endoscopically controlled work. The main issue is ergonomic: it is helpful to have an endoscope that stays out of the way so that other instruments can be used simultaneously. At minimum, an appropriately sized suction device is a necessary second instrument. If possible, 2 additional instruments offer greater surgical possibilities.

New technologies continue to improve the image produced by endoscopes. For example, with the appropriate endoscope, viewing apparatus, and image processing, a 3-dimensional image can be produced. The surgeon can then view the image with the aid of polarized glasses. As an alternative to standard-definition video, new high-definition images are available and more closely approximate the view that most neurosurgeons are familiar with from the operating microscope.

In addition to endoscopes, specialized instruments are helpful for minimally invasive cranial work, regardless of whether the work is performed with an endoscope or microscope. These instruments include narrow-shafted bipolar instruments; various slim dissectors; and single-shafted bayoneted scissors, pituitary forceps, and graspers. Angled dissectors, bipolar forceps, and a suction device that can operate around corners are highly advantageous. Without these instruments, the endoscope may reveal areas of residual tumor that remain out of reach due to the working angles available to straight-shafted instruments.

OPERATING TECHNIQUE

The principal issue for operating with the endoscope is maintaining the appropriate orientation. The novice endoscopist may find the view from the endoscope disorienting compared with the view provided by the microscope. This problem improves with experience. Familiarizing oneself with the endoscopic view during laboratory or practical courses is invaluable. Looking at known objects through the endoscope also can help one to adapt more rapidly to the endoscopic perspective.

In general, the endoscope is held in the nondominant hand and the working instrument or suction is held in the dominant hand. A 30° endoscope is most often used. This endoscope provides enough of an angle to be useful for looking around corners while still allowing the user to see straight ahead. Each time instruments are introduced into the field, the endoscope is removed so that the instruments can be followed into the head. This strategy prevents conflicts between the instruments and neurovascular structures.

The angled endoscope is readjusted alternately to inspect each direction where additional visualization is needed. Each time such an adjustment is made, the endoscope is withdrawn from the head, the angle is changed, and the endoscope is reinserted to prevent the tip from wandering into structures as the endoscope is rotated.

Tumor removal proceeds in a standard fashion, either with the use of the endoscope or with microsurgical instruments, such as scissors, a bipolar device, and dissectors. The endoscope is especially used at the end of surgery to check the completeness of resection and repair.

MINIMALLY INVASIVE CRANIOTOMIES

Various craniotomies are classified as keyhole approaches. The keyhole approach is usually defined by comparison to an alternative conventional craniotomy. For example, an eyebrow supraorbital craniotomy is a variation of the pterional or orbitozygomatic approach. A keyhole subtemporal approach is a variation of the traditional temporal approach. The important intellectual distinction between a conventional craniotomy and a keyhole approach is that in a conventional craniotomy, the size of the opening is typically larger than the target, with its circumference contracting as the depth of the approach increases. In a keyhole craniotomy, the surface opening can be smaller than the target, and the target is completely exposed by subtending different angles of approach (**Fig. 1**). Any approach may be made more minimally invasive by making an opening that requires the surgeon to take advantage of the various angles of view offered compared with a single trajectory. When no surface opening can expose the target without undue manipulation of neurovascular structures, the endoscope may offer additional opportunities for exposure.

The retrosigmoid approach is a common craniotomy that many neurosurgeons are familiar with as a keyhole approach. The surface opening is often modest because of the constraints of the local anatomy. The target is often deep. The cranial nerves are laid out in a "picket fence," that is, their exposure from top (usually the trochlear nerve) to bottom (spinal accessory nerve) can best be achieved by sweeping the view from one side to the other through the craniotomy. In the hands of many surgeons, only a very small craniotomy (often

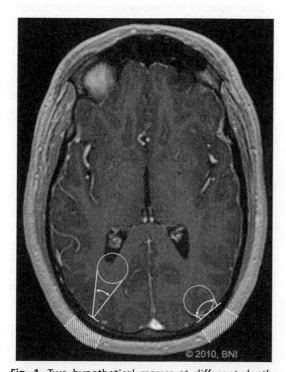

Fig. 1. Two hypothetical masses at different depths show the effect of depth on the cranial opening required. In the example on the left, the mass is deeply located and the craniotomy shown is therefore more than adequate to allow it to be exposed through a small cortical opening. Although the more superficial lesion located on the right is of the same size as the lesion on the left, full use of the same size craniotomy and an even larger cortical opening are needed. (*Courtesy of* Barrow Neurological Institute, Phoenix, AZ.)

of the order of 1 cm or slightly more) is necessary to expose this region.

Supraorbital Eyebrow Craniotomy for Tumors

Different names have been given to the craniotomy made through an incision in or around the eyebrow, such as the supraciliary, transbrow, transciliary, and supraorbital, among others.[3,4,30–34] Regardless of the name, it consists of an incision in the eyebrow through which a low frontal craniotomy is made, with or without removal of the orbital rim. The approach can be used to access the frontal pole, subfrontal region, suprasellar region, and retrosellar region. In most cases, the supraorbital approach can substitute for the orbitozygomatic approach and its variants.[4,34]

A prototypical tumor for which this approach can be considered is the craniopharyngioma,[35] for which various approaches have been applied. In general, a simple distinction determines the best route to the tumor. For retrochiasmatic and predominantly sellar or suprasellar tumors, the endonasal approach is preferred. For prechiasmatic tumors, a supraorbital eyebrow approach is usually preferred.[36–38]

Meningiomas, which involve neurovascular structures in the anterior cranial fossa, are usually best approached from above. The more posteriorly the meningiomas are located in the anterior cranial fossa, the more amenable they are to removal via an eyebrow approach because the olfactory groove tends to remain below the plane of the roof of the orbit, which may obstruct the access from an eyebrow craniotomy. If there is no attachment between a midline tumor and the anterior cerebral artery complex or optic nerves, the lesion also can be approached via an endonasal approach.

The access afforded by the eyebrow craniotomy is usually restricted to the anterior cranial fossa and to the structures immediately deep to the fossa in the upper basilar trunk and basilar cisterns. The incision cannot easily be extended laterally for these reasons: (1) the nature of overlying soft tissues, (2) a desire to avoid transecting too much of the temporalis muscle transversely, and (3) cosmetic concerns related to the consequences of sectioning the frontalis branch of the facial nerve. Therefore, the eyebrow craniotomy is not favored for lesions that fall below the sphenoid wing or that lie in the lower mesial temporal region. As noted, the olfactory groove can be accessed, but doing so is awkward at its most anterior reaches.

Transfalcine and Transtentorial Approaches

The principles of minimally invasive neurosurgery support not just smaller openings but also ones with less impact on neurovascular structures. For lesions located deep to the convexities of the skull and adjacent to the falx cerebri or tentorium, the option of crossing these structures has advantages. The patient should be positioned so that the brain on the side of the entry falls away from the dural fold by gravity so that gravity brings the target closer to the falx or tentorium. A small craniotomy then provides access to the gap between the brain and dural fold, and image guidance can be used to localize the lesion. The falx or tentorium can be opened and the lesion accessed, often without traversing any normal brain tissue (**Fig. 2**). Neuroendoscopy is often helpful for full evacuation of the extent of such resections, because the working angles are limited by the dura or by neurovascular structures that must be preserved.

Minimally Invasive Craniotomy for Removal of Intra-axial Brain Tumors

Minimally invasive craniotomies are well suited for addressing intra-axial pathologies. Regardless of its size, the deeper into the brain that any lesion lies, the smaller the arc that must be subtended to access it (**Fig. 3**). A larger craniotomy often merely exposes a larger area of the brain to potential harm. The chief concern is usually the brain tissue that must be transversed to reach the tumor, and this concern is the same for both minimally invasive craniotomies and conventional openings. The endoscope can be used to work within the cavity, allowing the surface opening to be even smaller.

To aid with exposure, various tubular retractors are available for access to deep tumors.[20,39] A tubular retractor has theoretical advantages because its placement should require a smaller scalp and bone opening and be less traumatic to transgressed brain tissue compared with the placement of conventional retractors. Tubular retractors also can facilitate the removal of intra-axial lesions in an endoscopically controlled fashion. Kelly and colleagues[40] pioneered the stereotactic tubular retractor system for resection of deep brain tumors. Otsuki and colleagues[41] described a method of using a similar retractor fixed to a Leksell stereotactic frame. The tube had a side port through which the instruments were placed for tumor resection. The investigators achieved gross total resection of 7 small lesions and partial resection of 8 larger lesions. Other

than transient aggravation of hemiparesis in 1 patient, there were no significant complications.

More recently, Kassam and colleagues[21] reported their results after intra-axial resection of 21 lesions, including 12 metastases, 5 glioblastomas, 3 cavernous malformations, and 1 hemangioblastoma, using only the endoscope. Gross total resection was achieved in 8 cases, near-total resection in 6 cases, and subtotal resection in 7 cases. There were no complications directly caused by the use of the endoscope and no postoperative hematomas, worsened neurologic deficits, or postoperative seizures. As the investigators discussed, there are 2 keys to resecting intra-axial lesions with the endoscope in this manner. First, the retractor must be dynamic and capable of being placed at multiple angles to see different views of the lesion. Second, the tubular retractor must be a conduit that allows bimanual use of instrumentation so that tumor can be resected using standard microsurgical techniques.

Similarly, Akai and colleagues[42] used a clear tubular retractor to remove intrinsic brain tumors from 3 patients. The tube was integrated with image guidance. The investigators were able to perform biopsy and coagulate tissue but noted that limitations associated with the instruments for coagulation limited the scope of what they could accomplish surgically. This point highlights that the evolutionary goal of minimally invasive approaches must be bimanual surgery with techniques that are equal to or better than traditional microsurgical techniques.

Although tubular retractors have their advocates, they are not entirely essential for endoscopically assisted minimally invasive resection of intrinsic tumors. In some cases, the working cavity is created as tumor removal proceeds. However, these studies do demonstrate that endoscopically controlled removal of intra-axial tumors is feasible in appropriately selected patients. Whether it will prove an improvement on prior techniques remains to be seen.

OUTCOMES

The literature on clinical outcomes after resection of intra- or extra-axial lesions of the cranium is sparse. Most data are in the form of case reports or small retrospective reviews. Given the paucity of conclusive outcome data, it is difficult to compare endoscopic neurosurgery with standard microneurosurgical techniques. To date, no studies have conclusively demonstrated the superiority of the endoscopic approach for tumor removal. Nevertheless, a review of the literature offers some insight into the progress of

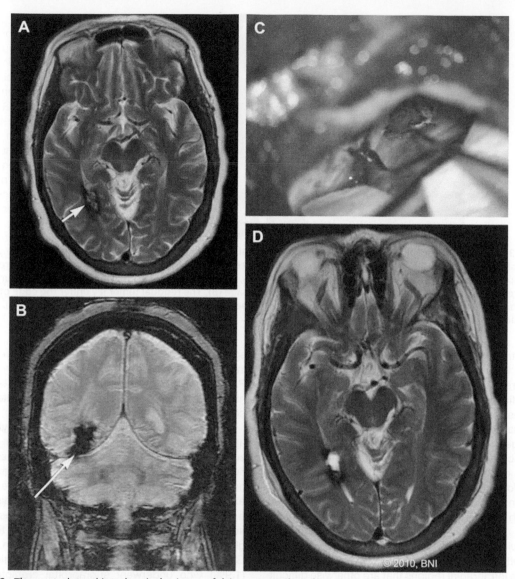

Fig. 2. The contralateral interhemispheric transfalcine approach and retrosigmoid transtentorial approaches take advantage of the natural space created between the brain and these fixed dural structures by gravity. In this example, a cavernous malformation medial to the ventricles is approached transtentorially to avoid harming the visual fibers. (*A*) Axial T1-weighted magnetic resonance (MR) image shows the lesion (*arrow*). (*B*) Coronal T2-weighted gradient-recalled echo MR image shows that the lesion reaches the tentorium. The trajectory to the lesion is shown with an arrow. (*C*) Still image from the intraoperative video shows the opening being made in the tentorium. (*D*) T2-weighted MR image shows the resection cavity of the cavernous malformation and preservation of the surrounding brain. (*Courtesy of* Barrow Neurological Institute, Phoenix, AZ.)

neuroendoscopic surgery and some of the successes and failures associated with the technique.

Many groups have published their experience with endoscopically assisted procedures. As mentioned, Fries and Perneczky[15] reported 380 cases of endoscopically assisted brain surgeries, which included 205 tumors. Excluding intraventricular and sellar lesions, the investigators

operated on 242 lesions in the brain parenchyma or subarachnoid space. Conclusions were primarily subjective evaluations of the utility of the endoscope in each case. Although there was no comparison group, Fries and Perneczky concluded that the endoscope decreased operating time because the visualization it provided precluded the need for more extensive dural and bony resection. Two cases were presented to

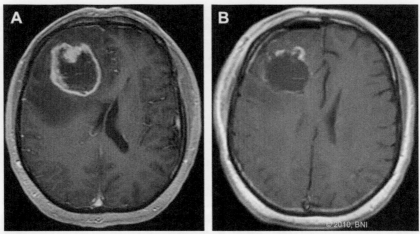

Fig. 3. Precautions for minimally invasive approaches. Axial T1-weighted magnetic resonance (MR) image with gadolinium shows a glioblastoma multiforme (*A*) approached through a small incision in a forehead crease. Removal of the bulk of the tumor was simple. Paradoxically, however, a small residual was missed on the surface nearest to the surgeon, as seen on the postoperative MR image (*B*). The residual tumor lay under the edge of the opening outside the view of the trajectory of the microscope. An endoscope with a highly oblique view (eg, 70°) would have been a useful adjunct in such a case. (*Courtesy of* Barrow Neurological Institute, Phoenix, AZ.)

illustrate this point. The investigators estimated that the time saved ranged from 10 minutes to 2 hours. Although there was no objective evidence confirming the benefit of the endoscope, the investigators demonstrated that the improved visualization can be valuable during intracranial surgery. Furthermore, there were no complications attributable to the endoscope. They described the use of the endoscope to visualize and preserve perforators during aneurysm surgery as well as to inspect tumor beds in deep-seated regions, such as the brainstem parenchyma, highlighting the potential improvement in visualization provided by the endoscope.

Others have reported similar benefits for visualizing intracranial regions that are otherwise difficult to access. Taniguchi and colleagues[43] reported 3 jugular foramen schwannomas that were removed primarily with the operating microscope. The endoscope was then used to visualize and resect residual tumor extending into the jugular foramen. Selvapandian[44] reported 4 cases of simultaneous thalamic glioma biopsy and cerebrospinal fluid diversion by ventriculostomy with no complications.

Complications

Complications of minimally invasive tumor neurosurgery are similar to those related to any standard craniotomy. Because the approaches are smaller and have more restricted working angles, concern is often raised about the risk of injury to neural or vascular structures caused by working in a small

space. However, at present there is little evidence in the literature for or against this proposition. Proper surgical planning and meticulous technique are the keys to obtaining a low rate of complications.

Specific complications associated with keyhole approaches have been documented. For the supraorbital eyebrow craniotomy, the small surgical field and technical difficulty often make adequate dural closure difficult. Consequently, extra emphasis should be placed on obtaining a good closure, especially a good primary closure, supplemented with the use of sealants or fibrin glue and pericranial flaps as needed. Warren and Grant[34] reported that only 2 of 105 patients (1.9%) who underwent supraorbital craniotomy experienced a cerebrospinal fluid leak.

The supraorbital eyebrow craniotomy also carries some risk of frontalis paresis related to retraction or section of the frontal branch of the facial nerve. This problem can be avoided by keeping the incision small and not extending it laterally over the keyhole region. Temporary paresis is common; however, in Warren and Grant's[34] series, only 2 patients experienced longstanding forehead asymmetry. Concerns about cosmesis are often cited by detractors of the eyebrow approach; however, the authors have found that the incision is actually favored by plastic surgeons and the cosmetic results are usually excellent.

Complications that arise during procedures involving the endoscope most often occur during introduction or lateral movements of the rigid scope within the surgical field. Focusing only on the endoscopic image can lead to neglect of the other instruments in the field and of the impact of the endoscope shaft on structures that the tip has already passed. If 2 surgeons are performing the procedure, it is imperative that 1 observes and be responsible for avoiding such injuries. Another possible solution, as suggested by Kassam and colleagues,[23] involves simultaneous visualization of the images from the endoscope and from the surgical microscope. The image from the endoscope can be placed in the ocular pieces of the microscope along with the image from the microscope so that the surgeon can constantly monitor the position of the endoscope shaft in the surgical field. However, for many practitioners, monitoring both images simultaneously is difficult.

To avoid causing trauma with a second instrument, the surgeon should maintain the habit of keeping all instruments in use within the view of the endoscope at all times. The endoscope should be withdrawn whenever the instrument is withdrawn and used to visualize the replacement of the instrument (**Fig. 4**).

As noted, the endoscope itself potentially presents the greatest danger to neurovascular structures. Endoscope-related trauma can be prevented by inserting and removing the endoscope in a straight line. The endoscope should not be swung side to side, particularly in the depth of a surgical field. Whenever the direction of view is altered, the endoscope should

only be rotated around its long axis. For major changes of orientation or trajectory, the endoscope should be removed from the cranium, the new direction chosen, and the endoscope reinserted.

With care and attention to these principles, injuries directly caused by the endoscope should be rare. In their series, Fries and Perneczky[15] noted no complications related to the use of the endoscope itself. With experience, operating under endoscopic visualization becomes quite natural. The image provided by modern high-definition endoscopes is excellent. Further, the use of a binocular 3-dimensional endoscope provides a view that appears more like the view from the microscope, offers improved depth perception, and may be associated with a shorter learning curve.

SUMMARY

The approaches discussed in this article are all refinements of standard or traditional approaches. At the conclusion of any tumor surgery, it behooves the neurosurgeon to examine the approach and ask whether a less-invasive approach would have been adequate. Conversely, it is fair to consider whether a smaller approach would leave the surgeon with fewer options. However, it is also important to ask whether the larger approach is associated with so much additional morbidity that its use cannot be justified. For many intrinsic tumors, only a small corticotomy is required, and a smaller bony opening actually prevents damage to the overlying brain. For extrinsic tumors, the route chosen depends mostly on tumor location and the tumor's relationship to intervening neurovascular structures.

Minimally invasive approaches are applicable to a broad range of intracranial tumors. Through the use of the keyhole concept and careful choice of trajectory, many tumors can be removed through a small craniotomy with fewer traumas to soft tissue and bone. The decision to use a minimally invasive approach must be individualized based on the patient and tumor. All cranial neurosurgeons should be familiar with the advantages and limitations of these approaches to use them where necessary. The addition of endoscopy can improve the removal of tumor and help protect neurovascular structures. The principles involved in using these techniques in brain tumor surgery are potentially applicable to almost all intracranial tumors and form an important part of the neurosurgical armamentarium.

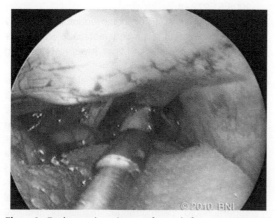

Fig. 4. Endoscopic view of a left retrosigmoid approach to the cerebellopontine angle. The endoscope is held in the right hand. A suction device is held in the left hand and kept in front of the endoscope so that it is in constant view to prevent inadvertent contact between the instrument and the cerebellum or cranial nerves. (*Courtesy of* Barrow Neurological Institute, Phoenix, AZ.)

REFERENCES

1. Jane JA, Park TS, Pobereskin LH, et al. The supraorbital approach: technical note. Neurosurgery 1982; 11:537–42.

2. Kaplan MJ, Jane JA, Park TS, et al. Supraorbital rim approach to the anterior skull base. Laryngoscope 1984;94:1137–9.

3. Jho HD. Orbital roof craniotomy via an eyebrow incision: a simplified anterior skull base approach. Minim Invasive Neurosurg 1997;40:91–7.

4. Reisch R, Perneczky A. Ten-year experience with the supraorbital subfrontal approach through an eyebrow skin incision. Neurosurgery 2005;57: 242–55.

5. Cappabianca P, Cinalli G, Gangemi M, et al. Application of neuroendoscopy to intraventricular lesions. Neurosurgery 2008;62(Suppl 2):575–97.

6. Walker ML. History of ventriculostomy. Neurosurg Clin N Am 2001;12:101–10, viii.

7. Dandy W. The brain. In: Lewis D, editor. Practice of neurosurgery. Hagerstown (MD): WF Prior Company; 1932. p. 247–52.

8. Guiot J, Rougerie J, Fourestier M, et al. [Intracranial endoscopic explorations]. Presse Med 1963;71: 1225–8 [in French].

9. Fukushima T, Ishijima B, Hirakawa K, et al. Ventriculofiberscope: a new technique for endoscopic diagnosis and operation. Technical note. J Neurosurg 1973;38:251–6.

10. Powell MP, Torrens MJ, Thomson JL, et al. Isodense colloid cysts of the third ventricle: a diagnostic and therapeutic problem resolved by ventriculoscopy. Neurosurgery 1983;13:234–7.

11. Caemaert J, Abdullah J. Endoscopic management of colloid cysts. Tech Neurosurg 1995;1:185–200.

12. Eiras AJ, Alberdi VJ. [Endoscopic treatment of intracranial lesions. Apropos of 8 cases]. Neurochirurgie 1991;37:278–83 [in French].

13. Lewis AI, Crone KR, Taha J, et al. Surgical resection of third ventricle colloid cysts. Preliminary results comparing transcallosal microsurgery with endoscopy. J Neurosurg 1994;81:174–8.

14. Perneczky A, Fries G. Endoscope-assisted brain surgery: part 1—evolution, basic concept, and current technique. Neurosurgery 1998;42:219–24.

15. Fries G, Perneczky A. Endoscope-assisted brain surgery: part 2—analysis of 380 procedures. Neurosurgery 1998;42:226–31.

16. Apuzzo ML, Heifetz MD, Weiss MH, et al. Neurosurgical endoscopy using the side-viewing telescope. J Neurosurg 1977;46:398–400.

17. Bushe KA, Halves E. [Modified technique in transsphenoidal operations of pituitary adenomas. Technical note (author's transl)]. Acta Neurochir 1978;41:163–75 [in German].

18. Jankowski R, Auque J, Simon C, et al. Endoscopic pituitary tumor surgery. Laryngoscope 1992;102: 198–202.

19. Jho HD, Carrau RL. Endoscopic endonasal transsphenoidal surgery: experience with 50 patients. J Neurosurg 1997;87:44–51.

20. Greenfield JP, Cobb WS, Tsouris AJ, et al. Stereotactic minimally invasive tubular retractor system for deep brain lesions. Neurosurgery 2008;63:334–9.

21. Kassam AB, Engh JA, Mintz AH, et al. Completely endoscopic resection of intraparenchymal brain tumors. J Neurosurg 2009;110:116–23.

22. Brown AP, Thompson BG, Spetzler RF. The two-point method: evaluating brain stem lesions. BNI Quarterly 1996;12:20–4.

23. Kassam A, Horowitz M, Welch W, et al. The role of endoscopic assisted microneurosurgery (image fusion technology) in the performance of neurosurgical procedures. Minim Invasive Neurosurg 2005; 48:191–6.

24. Gondim JA, Schops M, de Almeida JP, et al. Endoscopic endonasal transsphenoidal surgery: surgical results of 228 pituitary adenomas treated in a pituitary center. Pituitary 2010;13:68–77.

25. Cavallo LM, Prevedello DM, Solari D, et al. Extended endoscopic endonasal transsphenoidal approach for residual or recurrent craniopharyngiomas. J Neurosurg 2009;111:578–89.

26. Yano S, Kawano T, Kudo M, et al. Endoscopic endonasal transsphenoidal approach through the bilateral nostrils for pituitary adenomas. Neurol Med Chir 2009;49:1–7.

27. Nejadkazem M, Samii A, Fahlbusch R, et al. A simplified direct endonasal approach for transsphenoidal surgery. Minim Invasive Neurosurg 2008;51:272–4.

28. Jho HD, Alfieri A. Endoscopic endonasal pituitary surgery: evolution of surgical technique and equipment in 150 operations. Minim Invasive Neurosurg 2001;44:1–12.

29. Chang SW, Gore PA, Nakaji P, et al. Juvenile intradural chordoma: case report. Neurosurgery 2008; 62:E525–6.

30. Bhatoe HS. Transciliary supraorbital keyhole approach in the management of aneurysms of anterior circulation: operative nuances. Neurol India 2009;57:599–606.

31. Brydon HL, Akil H, Ushewokunze S, et al. Supraorbital microcraniotomy for acute aneurysmal subarachnoid haemorrhage: results of first 50 cases. Br J Neurosurg 2008;22:40–5.

32. Dare AO, Landi MK, Lopes DK, et al. Eyebrow incision for combined orbital osteotomy and supraorbital minicraniotomy: application to aneurysms of the anterior circulation. Technical note. J Neurosurg 2001;95: 714–8.

33. Shanno G, Maus M, Bilyk J, et al. Image-guided transorbital roof craniotomy via a suprabrow approach: a surgical series of 72 patients. Neurosurgery 2001;48:559–67.

34. Warren WL, Grant GA. Transciliary orbitofrontozygomatic approach to lesions of the anterior cranial fossa. Neurosurgery 2009;64:324–9.

35. Teo C. Application of endoscopy to the surgical management of craniopharyngiomas. Childs Nerv Syst 2005;21(8–9):696–700.

36. Fatemi N, Dusick JR, de Paiva Neto MA, et al. Endonasal versus supraorbital keyhole removal of craniopharyngiomas and tuberculum sellae meningiomas. Neurosurgery 2009;64:269–84.

37. Gardner PA, Kassam AB, Snyderman CH, et al. Outcomes following endoscopic, expanded endonasal resection of suprasellar craniopharyngiomas: a case series. J Neurosurg 2008;109:6–16.

38. Gardner PA, Prevedello DM, Kassam AB, et al. The evolution of the endonasal approach for craniopharyngiomas. J Neurosurg 2008;108:1043–7.

39. Ross DA. A simple stereotactic retractor for use with the Leksell stereotactic system. Neurosurgery 1993;32:475–6.

40. Kelly PJ, Goerss SJ, Kall BA. The stereotaxic retractor in computer-assisted stereotaxic microsurgery. Technical note. J Neurosurg 1988;69:301–6.

41. Otsuki T, Jokura H, Yoshimoto T. Stereotactic guiding tube for open-system endoscopy: a new approach for the stereotactic endoscopic resection of intra-axial brain tumors. Neurosurgery 1990;27:326–30.

42. Akai T, Shiraga S, Sasagawa Y, et al. Intra-parenchymal tumor biopsy using neuroendoscopy with navigation. Minim Invasive Neurosurg 2008;51:83–6.

43. Taniguchi M, Kato A, Taki T, et al. Endoscope assisted removal of jugular foramen schwannoma; report of 3 cases. Minim Invasive Neurosurg 2005;48:365–8.

44. Selvapandian S. Endoscopic management of thalamic gliomas. Minim Invasive Neurosurg 2006;49:194–6.

Minimally Invasive Surgery (Endonasal) for Anterior Fossa and Sellar Tumors

Timothy Lindley, MD, PhD[a], Jeremy D.W. Greenlee, MD[a],*, Charles Teo, MD[b]

KEYWORDS

• Endoscope • Endonasal approach • Meningioma
• Adenoma • Craniopharyngioma

HISTORICAL PERSPECTIVE

The primary goal of any surgical approach is to adequately visualize and treat the pathologic condition with minimal disruption to adjacent normal anatomy. During the past 200 years, rapid advances have been made in endoscope technology and instrumentation. In 1806, Philipp Bozzini demonstrated the use of a device consisting of a tube that was illuminated by a candle and mirror to visualize structures within the human body.[1,2] In the mid-1880s, the term endoscope was coined by the French urologist Antonin Jean Desormeaux.[1] One of the key limitations of early endoscopes was poor illumination. The invention of the incandescent light bulb by Thomas Edison in 1879, followed by the development of fiberoptic technology beginning in 1926 by John Logie Baird, paved the way for greatly improved illumination systems.[1] Revolutionary advances in rod-lens technology through the mid-1990s greatly expanded visualization. Finally, progress in video and display technologies has made it possible to view exquisite real-time images on large screens in high definition (HD) and, in some cases, in 3 dimensions, in addition to video documentation for teaching and cataloging purposes.

Whereas initial endoscopes were only used for visualization, concurrent advances were being made in the development of new instruments to allow endoscopic procedures to be performed as well. Maximilian Nitze was an early pioneer in endoscopic surgery. He published the *Textbook of Cystoscopy* in 1889 and was the first to use movable loops for urological procedures.[2] The subsequent development of microinstruments and electrocautery made a wide range of endoscopic procedures possible. Although pioneers in urology and otolaryngology made rapid advancements in endoscopic approaches, it was many years later before neurosurgeons began to recognize its potential for the treatment of pathologic conditions of the anterior skull base and sella.

The first steps toward the eventual development of endonasal endoscopic neurosurgery came with the early work by Harvey Cushing, demonstrating the feasibility of transsphenoidal techniques for resection of the sellar lesion. In the late 1800s, attempts made by other researchers to access the sella through subfrontal or temporal approaches were associated with high perioperative mortality rates, with some reports approaching 80%.[3] Cushing's technique required first

[a] Department of Neurosurgery, University of Iowa Hospitals and Clinics, 200 West Hawkins Drive, Iowa City, IA 52242, USA
[b] Centre for Minimally Invasive Neurosurgery, POW Private Hospital, Barker Street, Randwick, NSW 2022, Australia
* Corresponding author. Department of Neurosurgery, University of Iowa Hospitals and Clinics, 200 West Hawkins Drive, Iowa City, IA 52242.
E-mail address: jeremy-greenlee@uiowa.edu

Neurosurg Clin N Am 21 (2010) 607–620
doi:10.1016/j.nec.2010.07.010
1042-3680/10/$ — see front matter © 2010 Elsevier Inc. All rights reserved.

making a sublabial incision followed by exposing the submucosa and then resecting the nasal septum to allow direct access to the sphenoid sinus. The posterior wall of the sinus was opened with an osteotome to provide direct access to the sella. Between 1910 and 1925, Cushing used his transsphenoidal approach on 231 patients with a mortality rate of 5.6%. However, improvements in the safety and the greater exposure provided by intracranial approaches, compounded by problems with persistent spinal fluid leaks and meningitis, ultimately cooled the enthusiasm for the transsphenoidal approach, and the approach was all but abandoned.

However, one of Cushing's students, Norman Dott, recognized the advantages of the transsphenoidal approach and continued to refine this technique. Gerard Guiot, a French neurosurgeon who worked with Dott, was impressed by the approach and went on to perform more than 1000 transsphenoidal pituitary adenoma resections.[3] He and his fellow, Jules Hardy, further improved the technique. With the introduction of the operating microscope, Hardy reported his ability to treat pituitary adenomas, craniopharyngiomas, clival chordomas, and meningiomas with morbidity and mortality rates that were less than those of transcranial approaches.[4]

With the revival and increasing popularity of the transsphenoidal approach and the development of the modern endoscope, neurosurgeons in the 1970s began to merge these techniques. Early applications used endoscopes to augment traditional microsurgical approaches to allow visualization of structures that were not within the direct line of sight. Apuzzo and colleagues[5] provided some of the first reports using 70° and 120° endoscopes to inspect the sella after a traditional microsurgical transsphenoidal resection. Finally, in the 1990s, multidisciplinary teams including neurosurgeons and otolaryngologists began to report on purely endoscopic endonasal transsphenoidal approaches. In 1997, Jho and Carrau[6] first published their experience with endoscopic endonasal transsphenoidal surgery on 50 patients. Their results revealed the promise of minimally invasive endonasal neurosurgery and paved the way for broader applications of the technology. This article discusses the current state of minimally invasive endonasal techniques to address the pathologic conditions of the anterior cranial fossa and parasellar region.

ANATOMY

Detailed understanding of the normal anatomy is critical in any neurosurgical procedure; however, this fact becomes even more important with endoscopic approaches, in which one can easily become disoriented. Some of the key advantages of using an endoscope for transsphenoidal surgery are the ability to angle the view and inspect the tumor bed, and the superior illumination in a deep and dark cavity. This new degree of visualization is initially unfamiliar and can further contribute to surgeon disorientation. It is important to take full advantage of the improved visualization capability by having a detailed understanding of the anatomy of the sella and surrounding structures and to identify key landmarks early in the operation.

A careful review of preoperative imaging is crucial. Magnetic resonance imaging (MRI) provides critical details regarding the anatomy of both the lesion being addressed and the adjacent critical normal structures, such as the pituitary gland, carotid arteries, cavernous sinuses, and cranial nerves. Intrasellar lesions, such as pituitary adenomas or Rathke cleft cysts, can cause the sella to become greatly expanded. Also, as a sellar mass expands, the anatomy of the carotid arteries can become distorted. The cavernous portion of the carotid artery forms the lateral walls of the sphenoid sinus. In a recent cadaver study, the normal distance between the carotid arteries was 21 ± 2.5 mm.[7] However, there can be great variability in the course of the carotid artery, particularly if the artery is displaced or encircled by the lesion. In a study of normal specimens, an extreme medial course of the carotid artery was identified in 8% of cases (Fig. 1).[8] The flow voids of the carotid arteries are easily identified on T2-weighted MRI, and understanding the relationship of the carotid arteries with the lesion is critical in avoiding complications. Another key structure is the optic chiasm and optic nerves. As a sellar mass expands, the diaphragma sellae is forced upward and displaces the optic chiasm. The diaphragm can act as a barrier from the optic apparatus during the resection and can be observed to come into the operative field as the lesion is resected. Alternatively, suprasellar masses, such as craniopharyngiomas, can extend around the superior surface of the chiasm, making difficult a gross total resection via a transsphenoidal approach alone. It is important to recognize this relationship preoperatively to avoid injury to the optic apparatus during resection. Finally, the location of the remaining normal pituitary tissue should be determined on preoperative imaging. The normal pituitary is often identifiable on dynamic gadolinium-enhanced T1-weighted MR images. The pituitary gland takes up the gadolinium early in the postinjection phase whereas the adenoma

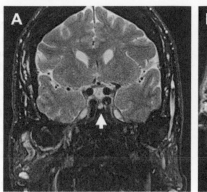
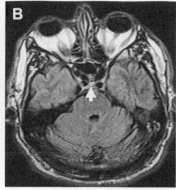

Fig. 1. Atypical anatomy of cavernous segment of carotid artery. As indicated by the arrows on the coronal T2-weighted magnetic resonance (*A*) and axial fluid-attenuated inversion recovery (*B*) images, this patient has unusually close cavernous carotid arteries. This variant must be recognized and considered when planning a trans-sphenoidal approach.

does not, and conversely, the gland shows no enhancement in the delayed scans whereas the adenoma does. Intrasellar masses often displace the normal pituitary posteriorly and to one side or the other. Understanding where the normal pituitary is located can help avoid intraoperative injury and prevent postoperative hormonal complications.

Whereas MRI provides important soft tissue detail, computed tomography (CT) provides information regarding the bony anatomy. The sphenoid sinus generally contains an intersinus septation (79% of cases)[8] and sometimes additional accessory septations. These septa most often terminate in the midline but can be present along the internal carotid artery prominence (26.7%) or along the optic prominence (19.6%).[8] Understanding the relationships between these septa and the carotid arteries preoperatively can help orient the surgeon (**Fig. 2**).

In addition, several bony landmarks can be identified intraoperatively. Typically, the carotid arteries and optic nerves are shielded by readily recognizable prominences along the roof and lateral walls of the sphenoid sinus. As the carotid artery prominence curves posteriorly along the lateral wall of the sinus, it passes just inferior to the optic nerve prominence. The depression just lateral to this junction is the lateral opticocarotid recess, which corresponds to the pneumatization of the anterior clinoid process. The prominent bulge between the carotid prominences is the sella. Identifying these structures early in the case is critical to remaining oriented, and frameless stereotaxy can be a helpful confirmatory adjunct (**Fig. 3**). An expansile mass can erode the overlying bone and obscure these landmarks, leaving them more susceptible to injury. In addition, bony dehiscences of the optic or carotid protuberances or anterior skull base are commonly identified on imaging, even without erosive pathologies. The presence of Onodi cells can also be identified on preoperative imaging, and these cells are present in approximately 8%

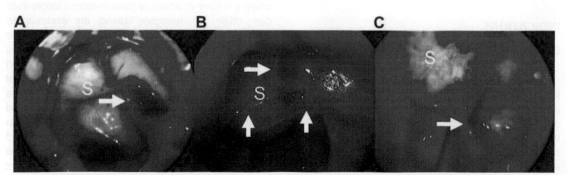

Fig. 2. Variations of septation encountered within the sphenoid sinus. (*A*) Paramedian vertical septation (*S*) attaching to the left carotid protuberance (*arrow*). (*B*) Complex 3-limbed vertical and horizontal septation (*arrows*). (*C*) Incomplete vertical midline septation (*arrow*).

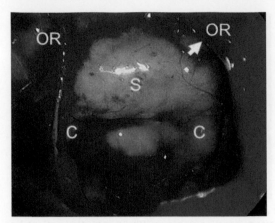

Fig. 3. Typical endoscopic view of posterior wall of sphenoid, with panoramic visualization of opticocarotid recesses (OR), sella (S), and carotid protuberances (C).

of cases.[8] Onodi cells are posterior ethmoid cells that can displace the sphenoid sinus posteriorly and interfere with the identification of common landmarks. More importantly, Onodi cells can contain the optic nerve, and it is important that these cells be recognized to avoid inadvertent optic nerve injury during ethmoidectomy.

Endonasal approaches were originally used to treat only sellar lesions, but now these approaches can be used to address a variety of midline skull base lesions. The nasally accessible boundaries extend from the cribriform plate anteriorly to the superior portions of the cervical spine posteriorly. The lateral boundaries are defined by the medial orbital walls anteriorly and the cavernous sinus and carotid arteries posteriorly. With proper training and experience, coupled with appropriate angled endoscopes and instruments, neuronavigation system, and preoperative planning, a wide variety of lesions can now be safely and successfully treated with the minimally invasive endonasal approach.

INDICATIONS

Endoscopic endonasal approaches to midline skull base lesions have several advantages when compared with traditional open approaches. The lesion can be directly accessed without retraction of the brain or neurovascular structures; the blood supply of the lesion can often be controlled early in the procedure; and visualization is improved, with better illumination, higher magnification, and a larger field of view than obtained by using the operating microscope. In addition, less morbidity, less blood loss, and shorter hospital stays have been reported with endoscopic approaches.[9]

However, several critical issues need to be considered when determining whether an endoscopic approach is appropriate for an individual patient. The goal of the surgery needs to be clearly defined because achieving it will ultimately determine a successful outcome. This consideration should be the same regardless of whether an endonasal endoscopic or open approach is used. For example, some lesions may be amenable to biopsy alone, whereas in other cases patients would be better served with subtotal or gross total resection.

If the goal of the procedure is to achieve a gross total resection, several anatomic relationships should be studied on preoperative imaging to determine if this goal is feasible. The degree of pneumatization of the sphenoid bone determines the size of the operative corridor and how readily identifiable the bony landmarks within the sphenoid sinus will be.[10] With a poorly pneumatized sphenoid sinus, the bone is thicker and superficial landmarks are more difficult to identify. Thus, more drilling will be required to gain adequate access and the risk of a complication may be higher.[10] Endoscopic approaches are ideally suited for midline lesions with minimal lateral extension. In general, lesions that extend laterally beyond the medial orbital walls invade the cavernous sinus and encircle the carotid arteries or infiltrate the bone and soft tissue of the face, and these lesions may be best treated with an open approach. The presence of brain invasion or extensive intradural involvement is also an important consideration that may lead one more toward an open approach. A cerebrospinal fluid (CSF) cleft on T2-weighted magnetic resonance image, the amount of brain edema, and the size of the mass can all aid in determining if brain invasion has occurred. The relationship of the mass with large arteries and the visual apparatus also needs to be studied carefully. Often, intrasellar lesions, such as pituitary adenomas, displace the carotid arteries laterally and the optic chiasm superiorly. Even when pituitary adenomas have become large, they can often be resected using an endoscopic approach. However, predominantly suprasellar lesions can displace or encircle the optic nerves, carotid arteries, and anterior cerebral arteries in such a way as to potentially cause the endonasal approach to be more difficult and potentially more morbid. Recurrent disease with fibrosis and destruction of normal anatomic landmarks can also be viewed as relative contraindications.[11] Finally, if an en bloc resection is desired based on oncologic principles, such as for nasopharyngeal carcinomas, an open craniofacial approach is likely to be superior because endoscopic resections are generally performed piecemeal.

PITUITARY ADENOMAS

Most of the early work demonstrating the promise of endonasal endoscopic surgery for anterior skull base lesions was performed by pioneers in pituitary surgery. Initially, the endoscope was used in conjunction with open microneurosurgical techniques. As surgeons became more comfortable with using the endoscope and as additional instrumentation was developed, it became possible to perform purely endoscopic resections with the goal of causing less damage to normal anatomy during exposure.[12] In 1992, Jankowski and colleagues[13] demonstrated the feasibility of performing purely endoscopic pituitary adenoma resections in their report on 3 patients. This report was followed by one by Jho and Carrau[6] in 1997, which described resection of pituitary adenomas by an endoscopic endonasal transsphenoidal approach in 44 patients. Of these patients, 13 had microadenomas, 16 had intrasellar macroadenomas, 9 had macroadenomas with suprasellar extension, and 6 had macroadenomas with invasion into the cavernous sinus. Among the patients with secreting tumors, 21 of 25 improved clinically. Of the 19 patients with nonsecreting adenomas, postoperative imaging revealed total resection in 16 and residual disease within the cavernous sinus in 3. More than 50% of the patients required an overnight hospitalization only, and all patients had clear nasal airways with minimal discomfort.

Since these early reports, large series have recently been reported, further verifying that pure endoscopic endonasal transsphenoidal resection of pituitary adenomas is a safe and effective procedure. Dehdashti and colleagues[14] reported on 200 patients with pituitary adenomas treated with purely endoscopic endonasal resection. Total resection was reported in 96% of the patients with suprasellar extension and 98% of those with intrasellar lesions. With regard to functioning adenomas, the investigators achieved remission rates of 71% for growth hormone–secreting, 81% for adrenocorticotropic hormone–secreting, and 88% for prolactin-secreting adenomas.[14] In the series by Gondim and colleagues[15] on 228 pituitary adenomas treated by a purely endoscopic approach, a gross total resection in 79% of all cases was achieved, with a remission rate of 83% for nonfunctioning and 76% for functioning adenomas. These cases were not further classified by cavernous sinus invasion or suprasellar extension. In addition, the tumors treated by Gondim and colleagues were larger than in most previous reports, which would also influence resectability.

It is controversial as to whether purely endoscopic resections are associated with lower complication rates than traditional microneurosurgical techniques. CSF leak and meningitis are the most common complications for transsphenoidal surgery, regardless of the approach. The rate of CSF leak and meningitis is comparable between endoscopic and microsurgical approaches at 1.5% to 3.5% and 0.5% to 1%, respectively.[14,16] The risk of permanent diabetes insipidus (1%–7.6%), pituitary insufficiency (3%–13.6%), visual loss (0%–0.9%), ophthalmoplegia (0%–0.9%), and death (0%–0.9%) are also similar between the approaches.[14,16] It does seem clear that the purely endoscopic approach causes less injury to nasal tissues, resulting in fewer nasal complications and improved nasal outcome.[17] Recognized nasal complications associated with microsurgical exposures include nasal septum perforation, saddle nose deformity, anesthesia of the upper lip and anterior maxillary teeth, fracture of the hard palate, anosmia, fracture of the orbit or cribriform plate, and bleeding (**Fig. 4**). In a review of 150 pure endoscopic transsphenoidal resections, 10% of the patients had hyposmia and 2% had anosmia, 0.7% had a serious postoperative bleeding complication, and no other nasal complications were recorded.[18] However, it has been argued that most patients recover quickly with few nasal complications after the microsurgical resections as well.[16] Identifying small differences in complication rates are not possible without large randomized trials. Nevertheless, published results confirm that the purely endoscopic endonasal approach for the treatment of pituitary adenomas is at least as safe and efficacious as microsurgical techniques, and can offer faster recoveries and return to normal lifestyle (**Figs. 5** and **6**).

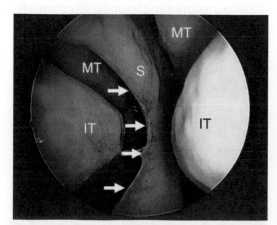

Fig. 4. Large nasal septal perforation (*arrows*) as a complication in a patient who was previously treated with a transseptal transsphenoidal surgery. IT, inferior turbinate; MT, middle turbinate; S, septum.

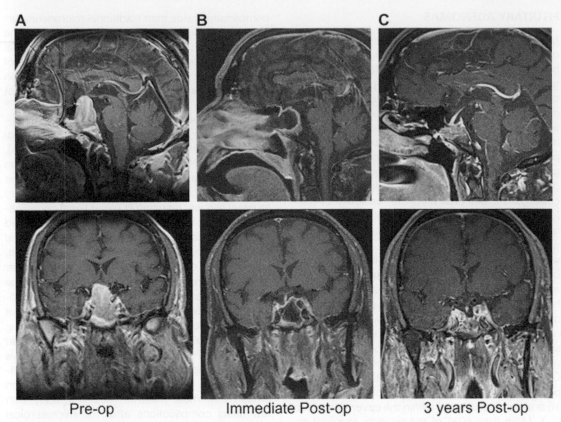

Fig. 5. Example case of a large pituitary adenoma with suprasellar as well as sphenoidal extensions before (*A*), immediately after (*B*), and 3 years after (*C*) endoscopic endonasal resection.

EXTENDED ENDOSCOPIC ENDONASAL APPROACH

Emboldened by the success of treating pituitary adenomas with an endonasal transsphenoidal approach and armed with new technology including improved endoscopes, neuronavigation

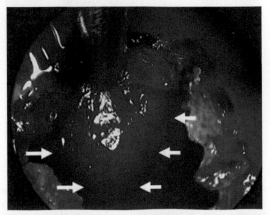

Fig. 6. Intrasellar view of normal pituitary gland (*arrows*) after excision of the adenoma.

systems, and specialized instrumentation, surgeons began seeking to expand the potential applications of this technology. Endoscopic endonasal approaches are now being used to treat a wide range of midline anterior skull base lesions. Dehdashti and colleagues[9] recently reported on the use of the endoscopic endonasal approach to treat 22 patients with lesions extending from the frontal sinus to the inferior clivus and foramen magnum. These lesions included 6 craniopharyngiomas; 4 esthesioneuroblastomas; 3 giant pituitary macroadenomas; 2 suprasellar Rathke pouch cysts; 2 angiofibromas; and 1 each of suprasellar meningioma, germinoma, ethmoidal carcinoma, adenoid cystic carcinoma, and suprasellar arachnoid cyst. Achieving a gross total resection is clearly more difficult in these complex cases than for typical pituitary adenomas, with a reported gross total resection rate of 73% for these diverse pathologies. However, the study highlights the ever-expanding indications for endoscopic endonasal skull base surgery.

The extended endonasal approach proves most advantageous in the treatment of skull base tumors in situations in which traditional open approaches are associated with significant morbidity. In particular, the authors discuss in greater detail the literature regarding the surgical management of particularly challenging anterior skull base pathologies, including craniopharyngiomas, tuberculum sellae meningiomas, and other more invasive tumors, including esthesioneuroblastoma and chordoma.

Tuberculum Sellae Meningiomas

Tuberculum sellae meningiomas provide a difficult surgical challenge owing to the density of the tumor tissue and adherence to vital structures including the anterior circulation arteries, pituitary gland and stalk, and cranial nerves. Classically, the pterional transsylvian approach is used, often in conjunction with an orbitofrontal osteotomy. An endonasal approach offers the opportunity to avoid potential cosmetic challenges, including postoperative enophthalmos, temporal wasting, and a large surgical scar, while also allowing for early obliteration of the tumor's vascular supply, thereby minimizing blood loss, and elimination of the need for brain retraction.

A detailed description of the endoscopic endonasal surgical approach has been recently reported.[19] One of the unique challenges to resecting tuberculum sellae meningiomas using an endonasal endoscopic approach is to first achieve adequate bony exposure of the ventral surface of the mass. The posterior border of the planum sphenoidale is identified by the sharp angle created at the junction with the anterior surface of the sella, while the medial opticocarotid recesses identify the lateral borders. After the mucosa is elevated, the bone is removed with a drill and rongeurs. Once the ventral surface of the mass is exposed, the ventral blood supply of the tumor can be obliterated with electrocautery. Being able to attack the blood supply of the mass early in the procedure allows for a near bloodless field. The dura can then be opened and the tumor debulked from within. After debulking the mass, the arachnoid plane around the tumor can typically be identified, and the lesion can be carefully dissected away from the ventral forebrain with no brain retraction. The magnified view that the endoscope provides allows for careful microdissection of the tumor capsule away from vital structures. After the mass has been resected, the anterior skull base is reconstructed using strategies described later.

de Divitiis and colleagues[19] reported their experience using the extended endoscopic transsphenoidal approach to treat 6 patients with tuberculum sellae meningiomas. Of these patients,

2 had tumors less than 2 cm in size and 4 had tumors 2 to 4 cm in size. A gross total resection was achieved in 5 patients. More than 90% of the tumor was resected in the sixth patient, who had residual tumor within the optic canal on postoperative imaging. Four of the patients who complained of preoperative visual deficits had complete resolution of their symptoms postoperatively. The complications cited included new diabetes insipidus in 1 patient and CSF leak in 2 patients; of these 2 patients, 1 ultimately had an intraventricular hemorrhage during the third revision of the leak repair and died. These results demonstrate the promise of the endoscopic endonasal approach and the importance of careful preoperative patient selection, and illustrate the importance of skull base reconstruction and dural repair.

An alternative minimally invasive approach for resection of tuberculum sellae meningiomas is the supraorbital craniotomy via an eyebrow incision. This technique is discussed in detail elsewhere in this issue. This method is effective to safely and completely remove these tumors, while still achieving excellent cosmetic results and minimizing recovery time. As such, surgeons have several good options as to which operation is likely to be the most effective and least morbid for each particular patient. A recent study that addressed this issue found that visual improvement and tumor extent of resection rates were similar between endonasal and supraorbital treatment groups; however, the complication rate was higher in the endonasal treatment group because of postoperative CSF leak.[20] These investigators suggest that tumors larger than 3 cm or extending beyond the supraclinoid carotid arteries should be approached via craniotomy (**Fig. 7**). The senior author (C.T.) uses the location of the anterior cerebral vessels as the main criterion for approaching these tumors from above or below. If there is a "cortical cuff" of gyrus rectus separating the posterosuperior dome of the meningioma from the anterior cerebral vessels, the authors favor an endonasal approach. Most olfactory groove and small tuberculum sellae meningiomas are grouped into this category. If the anterior cerebral vessels are intimately involved or indeed surrounded by tumor, a transcranial approach is recommended, of which the eyebrow minicraniotomy is the authors' preferred option.

Other reports do not separate supraorbital approaches from other transcranial approaches, but note similar results overall. For example, one series suggested a lower risk of visual worsening in patients treated with an endonasal approach compared with those treated transcranially.[21]

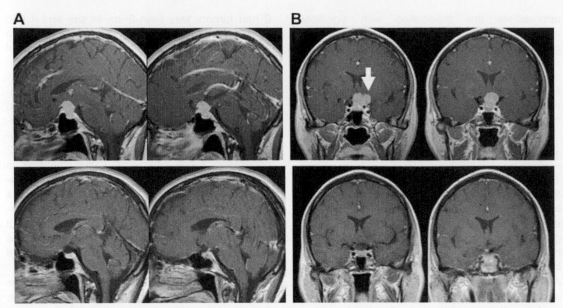

Fig. 7. Example case of tuberculum meningioma—which approach to use? This patient underwent a supraorbital craniotomy, given the lateral extent of the tumor (*arrow*). A complete excision was achieved as shown in the sagittal (*A*) and coronal (*B*) T1 postgadolinium images. Top row: preoperative; bottom row: postoperative.

These investigators, like Fatemi and colleagues,[20] further acknowledge the difficulties of skull base repair and CSF leak after an extended transsphenoidal resection. A different small case series reported improved visual acuity in patients treated with the endonasal approach compared with those treated with a transcranial approach, yet there was no difference in visual field outcomes between the different techniques.[22]

Craniopharyngioma

Craniopharyngiomas are neoplasms derived from squamous epithelial remnants of the Rathke pouch, and can have both sellar and suprasellar components. The extended endonasal approach allows for direct early tumor visualization without brain retraction. Further, these tumors often recur after initial subtotal resections. Reoperation, irrespective of the approach used, in this setting is treacherous because of arachnoidal scarring and gliosis with increased rates of incomplete resection and a higher complication rate.[23] [Teo CNS] For patients requiring re-resection, the transsphenoidal approach is particularly appealing because it allows for an unaltered path to the tumor in those patients who have previously undergone resection via craniotomy. Furthermore, many patients with recurrent tumors have panhypopituitarism, so the preservation of the pituitary gland and pituitary stalk are not concerns during transsphenoidal reoperation. Another factor that lends itself toward

endonasal treatment is a primarily retrochiasmatic tumor location (**Figs. 8** and **9**). These tumors, if approached via a subfrontal or transsylvian approach, require dissection around and under the optic nerves and chiasm, with the resultant risks of postoperative visual decline caused by manipulation or vascular compromise. The endonasal approach avoids such difficult dissection by its natural trajectory below and behind the optic apparatus, which is often elevated and displaced anteriorly by the tumor.

Cavallo and colleagues[23] described their experience using the extended endoscopic transsphenoidal approach to treat 22 patients who had previously undergone surgical resections of craniopharyngioma. A gross total resection was achieved in 9 patients and more than 95% of the tumor was resected in 8. Adherence to the optic nerves, perforating vessels, invasion of the hypothalamus, and parasellar or retroclival extension were identified as factors leading to a subtotal resection. Of 18 patients, 11 who had visual field deficits preoperatively experienced marked improvement and 6 reported that the defect normalized or had no change during follow-up, whereas 1 patient reported decreased vision in one eye and improvement in the other. CSF leak was reported in 13.6% of the patients. New-onset panhypopituitarism was identified in 2 patients. These results certainly compare favorably with the results of previous reports that used traditional open approaches.[24]

Pre-op   Immediate Post-op   9 mo Post-op

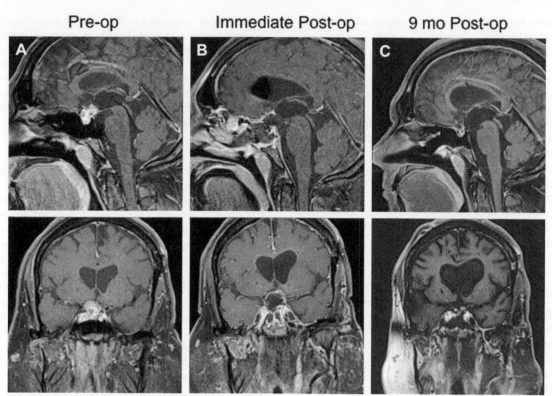

Fig. 8. Example case of a recurrent craniopharyngioma excised via an endoscopic endonasal approach. Column (*A*) shows preoperative images, column (*B*) shows immediate postoperative images demonstrating total resection, and column (*C*) shows images 9 months after surgery. Top row: sagittal T1 postgadolinium image; bottom row: coronal T1 postgadolinium image.

Like for tuberculum sellae meningiomas as discussed earlier, as well as for other suprasellar lesions, an alternative surgical option for craniopharyngioma removal is the supraorbital craniotomy. This minimally invasive approach is known to be safe and effective [Teo CNS], but

only a single case series compares this technique directly with endonasal approaches in a cohort of patients with craniopharyngioma.[20] These investigators found a greater extent of resection and improved visual outcome in the cohort of patients treated with the endonasal approach, and

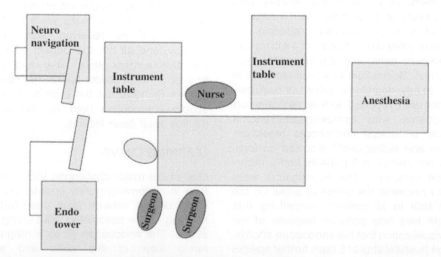

Fig. 9. Typical operating room setup for endoscopic endonasal surgery.

therefore recommended endonasal resection of retrochiasmal tumors over craniotomy. Conversely, the incidence of CSF leak and pituitary insufficiency was higher in patients treated with the endonasal approach than in those who underwent craniotomy. This series highlights the important considerations when choosing an approach for these difficult neoplasms, which are: lateral extent of the tumor—the more lateral the extent the more likely to approach the neoplasm transcranially; location of the chiasm—the more prefixed the more likely to approach transsphenoidally; preoperative hormonal and visual functions; and dural reconstruction. These issues require further study and additional case-control studies.

Esthesioneuroblastoma

Esthesioneuroblastomas are malignant sinus tumors arising from the olfactory epithelium. These invasive neoplasms typically involve the superior nasal vault and anterior skull base. The traditional surgical approach involves a craniofacial resection, which carries with it significant morbidity, including tension pneumocephalus, extra-axial fluid collections, anosmia, and frontal lobe retraction injury.

However, the midline location of these tumors and lack of intradural invasion has led investigators to explore the role of the endonasal endoscopic approach in resecting these complex lesions. Folbe and colleagues[11] described their multicenter results on 23 patients with esthesioneuroblastoma treated with this minimally invasive technique. Of these patients, 19 presented with primary disease and 4 had recurrent disease. All but one patient was treated successfully with a purely endoscopic approach, and 16 patients were treated with postoperative radiation. All patients with primary disease and 3 of 4 with recurrent disease were tumor free at a mean follow-up of 45.2 months. Spinal fluid leak was reported in 4 patients. No new neurologic deficits or perioperative fatalities were reported. In their recent report on 10 patients with esthesioneuroblastoma treated with endonasal endoscopic resection, Castelnuovo and colleagues[25] reported no local or regional recurrence in 9 patients and a recurrence in the neck in 1. The investigators were also able to preserve the sense of smell on the unaffected side in all patients, something that they thought was only possible because of the improved visualization that the endoscope affords. The average hospital stay of 5 days further speaks to the advantages of this less invasive approach.

Additional support for the use of endoscopic approaches for the treatment of esthesioneuroblastoma comes from a recent meta-analysis by Devaiah and Andreoli,[26] who reviewed the outcome data for 361 patients with esthesioneuroblastoma and found that endoscopic surgery compared favorably with open surgery in terms of survival for less invasive tumors.

Chordomas

Chordomas are another pathologic condition in which endoscopic endonasal approaches could greatly decrease the morbidity of resection. Chordomas are also discussed in another article elsewhere in this issue. Traditional approaches, including anterior transfacial, extended subfrontal transbasal, and lateral transtemporal approaches, are associated with significant morbidity. Hwang and Ho[27] described the use of the endoscopic endonasal approach coupled with neuronavigation to successfully treat 3 patients with large chordomas. Two of the patients underwent a single endoscopic procedure, and both were discharged home without complication on hospital day 3. The third patient had first undergone a craniotomy for resection of the superior portion of the mass and later underwent an endoscopic endonasal procedure to resect the residual inferior portion of the tumor. Fraser and colleagues[28] have subsequently reported their experience with endoscopic resection of chordomas in 7 patients. In 6 patients, a gross total resection was attempted. More than 95% resection was achieved in 5 patients, and 80% resection was achieved in the remaining case. One patient with multiple recurrent tumors underwent 2 intentionally subtotal palliative debulking procedures. No new neurologic deficits, intraoperative complications, or spinal fluid leaks were reported. Most of the patients received adjuvant radiation therapy, and all but the patient who underwent palliative surgery were alive and progression free at a mean follow-up of 18 months. These reports demonstrate the promise that the endoscopic approaches hold for the treatment of midline skull base lesions.

LEARNING CURVE

One of the major challenges that neurosurgeons face in performing purely endoscopic endonasal resections of anterior skull base tumors is the learning curve associated with using the endoscope. The endoscope gives a magnified panoramic view of the sella and surrounding structures; however, standard endoscopes only provide a 2-dimensional (2D) view, making depth perception difficult. This technical limitation along with the unfamiliar ergonomics of operating while looking up at a screen can also initially be awkward for surgeons who are used to standard bimanual microsurgical techniques. Furthermore, neurosurgeons have historically had limited training and exposure to basic handling and use of endoscopes. Thus, working with an experienced team of otolaryngologists who often use nasal endoscopy on a daily basis in clinic and surgery can shorten the learning curve of neurosurgeons acquiring new skills.[29] It is well documented that the complication rate decreases, the operative time decreases, and the extent of the resection increases as the surgeon becomes more familiar with the use of the endoscope.[18,30]

Recently, 3-dimensional (3D) endoscopes have been developed to provide improved depth perception and potentially shorten the learning curve for less experienced surgeons. Tabaee and colleagues[31] have described their experience using a 3D endoscope manufactured by Visionsense Ltd, Petach-Tikva, Israel, to perform 13 endonasal endoscopic transsphenoidal surgeries. The investigators have reported improved depth perception without physical discomforts, such as headache, nausea, or ocular fatigue. The authors have used a similar 3D endoscope and have had a similar experience.

TECHNICAL CONSIDERATIONS
Equipment

Multiple types of endoscopes and supporting equipment are commercially available for use in endoscopic endonasal surgery. Flexible or rigid endoscopes can be used. Rigid endoscopes are most commonly used because they are readily available in most hospitals, afford excellent high-resolution images, often in HD, are straightforward for surgeons to maintain and change viewing orientation, and can also serve as simultaneous intranasal retraction. The standard rod-lens endoscopes are available in several diameters and viewing angles. Typically, 0° and 30° optics are sufficient, but 45° or 70° optics are occasionally helpful. As the endoscope diameter decreases their fragility increases, and small telescopes (eg, 2 mm) can be easily damaged or broken entirely by improper handling or cleaning. The 4-mm-diameter, 18-cm-long telescopes afford excellent viewing image size, are robust to tolerate manipulation without breaking easily, are strong enough to retract structures such as the turbinates, allow excellent working space around the scope for other instruments, and do not block access to the nares. A lens cleansing or irrigating system (ie, sheath) is helpful to quickly clear blood or debris from the lens and increase efficiency.

Several manufacturers produce cameras that easily clip-mount to endoscopes, and there are options for standard or HD resolution. The same cameras can be used for other types of endoscopic surgery, such as thoracoscopy or laparoscopy, increasing the use and compatibility within hospitals. Likewise, light cables and sources are prevalent, interchangeable, and in some cases built into operating rooms. Standard liquid crystal display flat-screen monitors are used. Finally, a recording system or hard drive is helpful to save photographs and videos taken during surgery, for cataloging in the patient's medical record, for using for study purposes, or for instructional use. This equipment is ideally situated on a portable cart for easy transfer from one operating room to another, or can be boom-mounted within a given operating room to use space efficiently. Overall, viewing technology is advancing quickly, and video "chip-on-the-tip" scopes, smaller diameter scopes, and 3D systems are now being investigated.

Regarding surgical instruments, length, diameter, and physical size (ie, the ability of an instrument to fit in the endonasal corridor) are the only constraints to instrument suitability in endonasal surgery. Therefore, many standard microneurosurgical instruments can be used. However, because the view from endoscopes is at the tip and working instruments are passed along the shaft of the endoscope, bayoneted instruments are not required. In fact, straight instruments are preferred because they allow 360° rotation and tip usability without the bayoneted shaft impeding or affecting an adjacent instrument. This fact also obviates the need and expense of having multiple "right-" and "left-" or "up-" and "down-" angled instrument tips relative to the shaft.

Nevertheless, there are shortcomings in endonasal surgical instrumentation. Specifically, the ability to suture is extremely difficult. In addition, standard bipolar forceps are fairly ineffective and difficult to use because of their size and the tips being forced closed or prevented from opening by the surgical corridor. Longer and thinner diameter forceps are available, but these are limited by scissoring of the tips. Pistol-grip bipolar forceps are being developed to circumvent these problems, but they still require refinement.

Neuronavigation

Nowhere is it more critical to have a clear understanding of the relevant anatomy than during extended endonasal endoscopic surgery. Poor sphenoid sinus pneumatization or distortion of the anatomy from an expansile mass can further complicate the anatomy. Modern systems allow for navigation to be based off CT images to allow for high resolution of bony anatomy and on MR images to detail soft tissue and vascular structures. Neuronavigation can provide critical information before beginning the exposure to allow precise identification of the carotid arteries and optic nerves. The tumor margins can also be identified early in the case. This information allows for a wide bony exposure with less chance of injuring vital structures. Further, because most lesions treated using the endoscopic approach are intimately associated with the skull base, brain shift during surgery has little impact on the accuracy of neuronavigation during the procedure, improving its usefulness during tumor resection. Thus, neuronavigation should be routinely used in extended endonasal endoscopic cases.

Basic Operating Room Setup

Proper setup of the operating environment is important for effective and comfortable endonasal surgery. Of utmost importance are positions of viewing screens such that they can all be viewed comfortably from the surgeons' working position. As illustrated in **Fig. 9**, the endoscope screen and neuronavigation system are behind the patient's head to allow straight-on viewing by the surgical team. The scrub nurse should be directly opposite the surgeon to facilitate instrument transfer without the surgeon having to look away from the screen. The patient's head can be tilted away from and rotated toward the surgeon to aid access to the nares and improve surgeon comfort.

SPHENOIDAL APPROACH

The endonasal approach to the sphenoid sinus can be accomplished using a unilateral or bilateral nares technique. The binaris approach generally affords an improved opportunity for the surgeon to work using a bimanual method. This approach is recommended when first learning, for complex tumors requiring extended transsphenoidal approaches, and for moderate- and larger-size tumors.

The usual endonasal approach begins with mucosal decongestion using topical cocaine or oxymetazoline-soaked cottonoids followed by sphenopalatine blocks using local anesthetics. Next, the middle turbinates can be lateralized or partially resected depending on the surgeon's preference. This step allows visualization of the natural sphenoid ostia, which can be entered and enlarged. The overlying mucosa can be resected with oscillating debriders, while rongeurs or a drill can be used for bony removal of the anterior sphenoid. In addition, a partial posterior septectomy can be performed to facilitate bilateral access into the sphenoid sinus. The sphenoidotomy should be large, such that multiple instruments and the endoscope itself can be passed through the sphenoidotomy without being forced against each other by the bony edges of the remaining anterior sphenoid bone.

The sella and parasellar bony structures are immediately evident on entering the sphenoid sinus. At this point, the operative techniques for an endoscopic endonasal approach are the same as those for microsurgical approaches. In brief, intrasphenoidal septations should be taken down with a drill or rongeurs to complete the sellar exposure. Normal landmarks should be identified and confirmed as needed with neuronavigation. The mucosa overlying the bony entry point (eg, the midline sella for a pituitary tumor) is opened and cauterized to expose the bony anterior face of the sella. Because the sella is often enlarged by slow growing macroadenomas, bony defects are often seen after the mucosa is opened. If no defect is present, an opening can be created with a curet, drill, or small osteotome. The bony opening is then enlarged with rongeurs or a drill to extend from the ipsilateral carotid protuberance to the contralateral carotid protuberance, and from the floor of the sella to the planum sphenoidale inferosuperiorly. The dura is incised, and tumor debulking is performed with ring curettes, followed by a capsular dissection if possible. The normal pituitary gland should be preserved if possible.

CLOSURE TECHNIQUES

One challenging aspect of endoscopic endonasal surgery is achieving an adequate dural repair to prevent postoperative CSF leaks, which is particularly true when more complex extended endonasal procedures are attempted and bony and dural openings are larger. Several techniques have been described and are briefly reviewed here. After resection has been completed and hemostasis assured, a piece of collagen matrix or dural substitute is placed on the diaphragma sellae. A fat graft is then lodged within the dural defect such that a portion of the graft is intradural.[32] Some researchers advocate repairing the sella with autogenous bone graft.[30] The bone can be collected from the rostrum of the sphenoid, middle turbinate, or sphenoid septum, and this bone will support the fat graft. Alternatively, a sealant or tissue glue may be used. Anterior support of the dural repair may be achieved by sphenoidal packing with fat or cellulose sponges.

In cases in which a large dural defect is encountered intraoperatively or a postoperative CSF leak occurs, additional strategies have been suggested. One approach is to create a pedicled nasal septal flap based on the posterior nasal artery.[33] The flap can be positioned over the fat graft and then secured with tissue glue/sealant. The closure can be held in place with Nasopore sponges (Stryker, Kalamazoo, MI, USA) and a Foley catheter balloon. The balloon can be removed 3 to 5 days after surgery.[33] Finally, a novel technique has been reported to allow for creation of an endoscopically harvested vascularized pericranial flap that can be used to repair anterior skull base defects.[34] Two small incisions are made behind the hairline and a third along the natural skin crease of the glabella. The pericranial flap is created and passed inferiorly. After a small nasal osteotomy is created through the glabellar incision, the flap is passed into the nasal cavity. The vascularized pericranial flap is then positioned over the defect. Any time there is concern for a CSF leak, a lumbar drain can be placed and maintained for several days.

SUMMARY

As technological advancements in endoscope technology and neuronavigation systems have made their way into the operating room, investigators have only recently begun to discover the true potential of the extended endonasal endoscopic approach for anterior skull base lesions. With improved visualization, less brain retraction, and the promise of less morbidity than traditional open approaches, the indications will certainly continue to expand as surgeons gain experience and comfort with these new techniques. Further studies are required to more clearly identify factors influencing patient selection and to compare the long-term outcomes of endoscopic endonasal surgery with craniotomy for these expanding applications.

REFERENCES

1. Doglietto F, Prevedello DM, Jane JA Jr, et al. Brief history of endoscopic transsphenoidal surgery—from Philipp Bozzini to the First World Congress of Endoscopic Skull Base Surgery. Neurosurg Focus 2005;19(6):E3.

2. Mouton WG, Bessell JR, Maddern GJ. Looking back to the advent of modern endoscopy: 150th birthday of Maximilian Nitze. World J Surg 1998;22(12):1256–8.

3. Liu JK, Das K, Weiss MH, et al. The history and evolution of transsphenoidal surgery. J Neurosurg 2001;95(6):1083–96.

4. Hardy J, Robert F. [A meningioma of the sella turcica, subdiaphragmatic variety. Exeresis through the transsphenoidal route]. Neurochirurgie 1969;15(7):535–43 [in French].

5. Apuzzo ML, Heifetz MD, Weiss MH, et al. Neurosurgical endoscopy using the side-viewing telescope. J Neurosurg 1977;46(3):398–400.

6. Jho HD, Carrau RL. Endoscopic endonasal transsphenoidal surgery: experience with 50 patients. J Neurosurg 1997;87(1):44–51.

7. Unlu A, Meco C, Ugur HC, et al. Endoscopic anatomy of sphenoid sinus for pituitary surgery. Clin Anat 2008;21(7):627–32.

8. Unal B, Bademci G, Bilgili YK, et al. Risky anatomic variations of sphenoid sinus for surgery. Surg Radiol Anat 2006;28(2):195–201.

9. Dehdashti AR, Ganna A, Witterick I, et al. Expanded endoscopic endonasal approach for anterior cranial base and suprasellar lesions: indications and limitations. Neurosurgery 2009;64(4):677–87 [discussion: 687–9].

10. Cavallo LM, de Divitiis O, Aydin S, et al. Extended endoscopic endonasal transsphenoidal approach to the suprasellar area: anatomic considerations—part 1. Neurosurgery 2007;61(Suppl 3):24–33 [discussion: 33–4].

11. Folbe A, Herzallah I, Duvvuri U, et al. Endoscopic endonasal resection of esthesioneuroblastoma: a multicenter study. Am J Rhinol Allergy 2009;23(1):91–4.

12. Teo C, Dornhoffer J, Hanna E, et al. Application of skull base techniques to pediatric neurosurgery. Childs Nerv Syst 1999;15(2–3):103–9.

13. Jankowski R, Auque J, Simon C, et al. Endoscopic pituitary tumor surgery. Laryngoscope 1992;102(2):198–202.

14. Dehdashti AR, Ganna A, Karabatsou K, et al. Pure endoscopic endonasal approach for pituitary adenomas: early surgical results in 200 patients and comparison with previous microsurgical series. Neurosurgery 2008;62(5):1006–15 [discussion: 1015–7].

15. Gondim JA, Schops M, de Almeida JP, et al. Endoscopic endonasal transsphenoidal surgery: surgical results of 228 pituitary adenomas treated in a pituitary center. Pituitary 2010;13(1):68–77.

16. Fatemi N, Dusick JR, de Paiva Neto MA, et al. The endonasal microscopic approach for pituitary adenomas and other parasellar tumors: a 10-year experience. Neurosurgery 2008;63(4 Suppl 2):244–56 [discussion: 256].

17. Graham SM, Iseli TA, Karnell LH, et al. Endoscopic approach for pituitary surgery improves rhinologic outcomes. Ann Otol Rhinol Laryngol 2009;118(9):630–5.

18. Charalampaki P, Ayyad A, Kockro RA, et al. Surgical complications after endoscopic transsphenoidal pituitary surgery. J Clin Neurosci 2009;16(6): 786–9.

19. de Divitiis E, Cavallo LM, Esposito F, et al. Extended endoscopic transsphenoidal approach for tuberculum sellae meningiomas. Neurosurgery 2007;61(5 Suppl 2):229–37 [discussion: 237–8].

20. Fatemi N, Dusick JR, de Paiva Neto MA, et al. Endonasal versus supraorbital keyhole removal of craniopharyngiomas and tuberculum sellae meningiomas. Neurosurgery 2009;64(5 Suppl 2):269–84 [discussion: 284–6].

21. de Divitiis E, Esposito F, Cappabianca P, et al. Tuberculum sellae meningiomas: high route or low route? A series of 51 consecutive cases. Neurosurgery 2008;62(3):556–63 [discussion: 556–63].

22. Kitano M, Taneda M, Nakao Y. Postoperative improvement in visual function in patients with tuberculum sellae meningiomas: results of the extended transsphenoidal and transcranial approaches. J Neurosurg 2007;107(2):337–46.

23. Cavallo LM, Prevedello DM, Solari D, et al. Extended endoscopic endonasal transsphenoidal approach for residual or recurrent craniopharyngiomas. J Neurosurg 2009;111(3):578–89.

24. Jung TY, Jung S, Choi JE, et al. Adult craniopharyngiomas: surgical results with a special focus on endocrinological outcomes and recurrence according to pituitary stalk preservation. J Neurosurg 2009;111(3):572–7.

25. Castelnuovo P, Bignami M, Delu G, et al. Endonasal endoscopic resection and radiotherapy in olfactory neuroblastoma: our experience. Head Neck 2007; 29(9):845–50.

26. Devaiah AK, Andreoli MT. Treatment of esthesioneuroblastoma: a 16-year meta-analysis of 361 patients. Laryngoscope 2009;119(7):1412–6.

27. Hwang PY, Ho CL. Neuronavigation using an image-guided endoscopic transnasal-sphenoethmoidal approach to clival chordomas. Neurosurgery 2007; 61(5 Suppl 2):212–7 [discussion: 217–8].

28. Fraser JF, Nyquist GG, Moore N, et al. Endoscopic endonasal transclival resection of chordomas: operative technique, clinical outcome, and review of the literature. J Neurosurg 2010;112(5):1061–9.

29. Har-El G. Endoscopic transnasal transsphenoidal pituitary surgery—comparison with the traditional sublabial transseptal approach. Otolaryngol Clin North Am 2005;38(4):723–35.

30. Koc K, Anik I, Ozdamar D, et al. The learning curve in endoscopic pituitary surgery and our experience. Neurosurg Rev 2006;29(4):298–305 [discussion: 305].

31. Tabaee A, Anand VK, Fraser JF, et al. Three-dimensional endoscopic pituitary surgery. Neurosurgery 2009;64(5 Suppl2):288–93 [discussion: 294–5].

32. Ceylan S, Koc K, Anik I. Extended endoscopic approaches for midline skull-base lesions. Neurosurg Rev 2009;32(3):309–19 [discussion: 318–9].

33. El-Sayed IH, Roediger FC, Goldberg AN, et al. Endoscopic reconstruction of skull base defects with the nasal septal flap. Skull Base 2008;18(6):385–94.

34. Zanation AM, Snyderman CH, Carrau RL, et al. Minimally invasive endoscopic pericranial flap: a new method for endonasal skull base reconstruction. Laryngoscope 2009;119(1):13–8.

Expanded Endonasal Approaches to Middle Cranial Fossa and Posterior Fossa Tumors

Daniel M. Prevedello, MD[a],*, Leo F.S. Ditzel Filho, MD[b],
Domenico Solari, MD[b,c], Ricardo L. Carrau, MD[b],
Amin B. Kassam, MD[b]

KEYWORDS

- Endoscope • Skull base tumors • Meckel cave
- Posterior fossa • Middle fossa • Endonasal
- Extended transphenoidal • Expanded endoscopic approach

During the past decade, the increasing use of endoscopy in skull base surgery has become an important alternative to traditional transcranial surgery. Anatomic studies coupled with technological advances in endoscopic equipment, surgical instruments, and neurophysiological monitoring have allowed novel and exciting approaches to flourish within the field.[1–6] What once was only a route to the pituitary gland and sellar region has become a major highway to the entire ventral skull base and craniocervical junction.[6–14]

Among these innovations stand the expanded endonasal approaches (EEAs). The philosophy behind these approaches is, as in any skull base approach, to tailor the bone removal to gain a direct access to deep regions, thus minimizing manipulation of the cerebrum, blood vessels, and cranial nerves. Although deemed minimally invasive, these techniques provide a wide exposure of the cranial base and its pathologic conditions, often with early control of tumor-nurturing vessels and minimal or no neural tissue retraction.

Furthermore, minimally invasive must not be perceived as less effective but rather as a less-aggressive pathway to reach maximum effectiveness.

The EEA to the anterior cranial fossa and sellar/parasellar regions has already been well described and thus it is not discussed in this article.[6,10,13,15,16] Hence, the authors focus on EEA to the middle cranial fossa (MCF) and posterior fossa (PF).

MIDDLE CRANIAL FOSSA

Traditionally, neurosurgical procedures for the pathologic conditions of the MCF have been performed through lateral craniotomies. Although lesions located at the most lateral aspect of the temporal fossa are directly reached when a lateral approach is used, more medially located mass lesions require various degrees of temporal lobe manipulation and/or retraction. In this article, the endonasal route is presented as an alternative direct approach to the medial compartment of the MCF.

[a] Department of Neurological Surgery, The Ohio State University, 410 West 10th Avenue, Columbus, OH, USA
[b] Neuroscience Institute & Brain Tumor Center, John Wayne Cancer Institute at Saint John's Health Center, 2200 Santa Monica Boulevard, Santa Monica, CA 90404, USA
[c] Division of Neurosurgery, Department of Neurological Sciences, Università degli Studi di Napoli Federico II, Via Sergio Pansini, 580131, Naples, Italy
* Corresponding author. Department of Neurological Surgery, The Ohio State University, N-1011 Doan Hall, 410 West 10th Avenue, Columbus, OH 43210-1240.
E-mail address: dprevedello@gmail.com

Neurosurg Clin N Am 21 (2010) 621–635
doi:10.1016/j.nec.2010.07.003

Indications

Virtually any pathologic process can be accessed through an endonasal route as long as it is located in the medial portions of the middle fossa, dislocating the temporal lobe superolaterally. Several pathologic processes commonly arise in the middle fossa and can be directly reached through an EEA. Of special interest are meningiomas and trigeminal nerve schwannomas. Chordomas and chondrosarcomas can also extend cranially to the middle fossa when they grow to large sizes (**Fig. 1**). Juvenile angiofibromas grow from the pterygopalatine fossa (PPF) and can expand posteriorly into the middle fossa as well. Aggressive pituitary adenomas can also grow laterally into

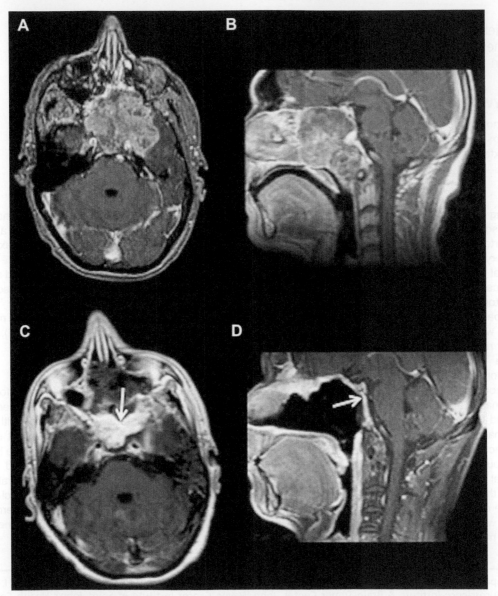

Fig. 1. (*A*) Axial and (*B*) sagittal preoperative magnetic resonance images showing a large clival chordoma in a 41-year-old male patient, which demonstrates heterogeneous enhancement after intravenous contrast injection. This tumor involves the entire midline, extending anteroposteriorly from the posterior portion of the nasal cavities to the clival area and rostrocaudally down to the nasopharynx at the level of the C1-C2 junction, also invading the left cavernous sinus and reaching the ipsilateral MCF. (*C*) Axial and (*D*) sagittal postoperative magnetic resonance images after an endoscopic endonasal approach, demonstrating the complete removal of the lesion. The arrows indicate the enhancing nasoseptal flap that has been used to reconstruct the skull base defect.

the cavernous sinus and Meckel cave. Sinonasal malignancies such as adenoid cystic carcinomas can infiltrate perineural tissue and use it as a gateway to reach the middle fossa. All these pathologic conditions are examples of diseases in which the endonasal route can facilitate resection without brain retraction.

Anatomic Considerations

To access the MCF through an endonasal corridor, one needs to completely understand the ventral cranial base anatomy.

The sphenoid sinus lateral recess is a pneumatized projection of the sinus under the middle fossa. Once the bone that covers the lateral wall of the sphenoid sinus is removed, the periosteum of the middle fossa is exposed. The meningeal layer of the dura is located lateral to the gasserian ganglion.

Meckel cave is basically a small compartment within the 2 layers of dura mater on the anteromedial portion of the MCF containing the trigeminal (gasserian) ganglion. The limits of the Meckel cave include the periosteal dural layer that covers the MCF bone at its medial and inferior aspect and the dural meningeal layer at its lateral and superior aspect that separates it from the subarachnoid space. From the gasserian ganglion, arise the 3 trigeminal branches: ophthalmic (V1), maxillary (V2), and mandibular (V3) nerves (**Fig. 2**A). The 3 nerves exit the skull through the superior orbital fissure (SOF), foramen rotundum, and foramen ovale, respectively.

The gasserian ganglion guards the MCF medially. While dealing with benign disease, the trigeminal nerve must be preserved. The pathway to reach the MCF from the sphenoid sinus is through the 2 anterior triangles of the cavernous sinus: the anteromedial and anterolateral triangles (see **Fig. 2**B). The anteromedial cavernous sinus triangle is limited superiorly by the ophthalmic branch of the trigeminal nerve (V1), pointing toward the SOF, and inferiorly by the maxillary branch (V2). On the other hand, the anterolateral triangle is enclosed within V2 superiorly and the mandibular branch (V3) inferolaterally. After bone removal, the exploration of these spaces allows the direct exposure of the temporal meningeal dura, which if needed can be followed posteriorly into the lateral component of Meckel's cave or opened laterally into the subarachnoid space.

The concept of the quadrangular space (QS) is important to deal with gasserian ganglion disease or pathologic conditions located medial to it. This "window" is bordered by the sixth cranial nerve (abducens nerve) superiorly, the maxillary branch

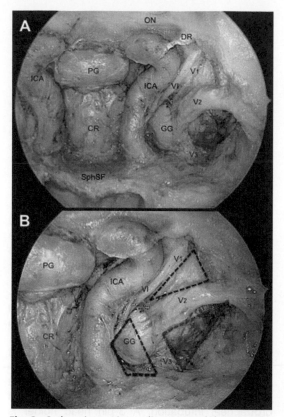

Fig. 2. Cadaveric specimen dissections. (*A*) Panoramic view of a wide opening of the sphenoid sinus with extensive bone removal of the anteromedial wall of the MCF, with exposure of the clival recess (CR), gasserian ganglion (GG) and the 3 trigeminal branches (V1, V2, and V3), internal carotid arteries (ICAs), and pituitary gland (PG). DR, proximal dural ring; ON, optic nerve; Sph SF, sphenoid sinus floor. (*B*) Panoramic view of the anterior left MCF with a 45° endoscope after bone removal. Of particular importance is the quadrangular space (*blue shaded line*), the anteromedial triangle (*black shaded line*), and the anterolateral triangle (*red shaded line*). VI, abducens nerve.

of the trigeminal nerve (V2) laterally, and the internal carotid artery (ICA) medially and inferiorly (see **Fig. 2**B).[12]

Appreciation of the sixth cranial nerve anatomy is also important for this approach, particularly its trajectory within the cavernous sinus. The sixth cranial nerve pierces the clival dura posterior to the ICA and advances between the dural layers superolaterally toward Dorello canal. Once inside the cavernous sinus, the nerve runs parallel to V1 on its way to the SOF. As the nerve ascends to the SOF, it forms the superior limit of the QS. The abducens nerve must be carefully observed and avoided during the approach to prevent undesirable postoperative sixth nerve palsy.

The medial and inferior aspects of the QS are created by the paraclival (vertical) and petrous (horizontal) portions of the ICA, respectively. Identification of these portions, particularly the paraclival segment, is essential for the proper exposure of the QS. The vidian nerve, formed by the union of the greater superficial petrosal nerve and the deep petrosal nerve, is used as a landmark for identification of the ICA anterior genu, where the petrous ICA turns into paraclival ICA at the foramen lacerum.

Surgical Technique

Preoperatively, computed tomography and magnetic resonance imaging of the head are carried out. Results of both the techniques are combined and fused for comprehensive intraoperative image guidance.

All EEAs are performed with cranial nerve monitoring (using electromyography), with special attention to the third, fourth, motor V3, and sixth cranial nerves ipsilateral to the disease. Also, somatosensory evoked potentials are monitored throughout the surgical procedure.

Once in the operating room, the patient undergoes standard intravenous anesthesia and orotracheal intubation. A 3-pin head holder is placed with a slight neck extension and discreet head rotation to the right and a tilt to the left.

The nasal cavity is decongested with topical 0.05% oxymetazoline; antisepsis is achieved with perinasal and periumbilical povidone solution (in case a fat graft is needed). Intravenous antibiotic, a third- or fourth-generation cephalosporin, is administered at the beginning of the procedure.

The procedure begins with the use of a 0°-lens endoscope. Initially, the inferior turbinates are displaced laterally. Next, the middle turbinate that is ipsilateral to the lesion is removed and its pedicle, a direct branch of the sphenopalatine artery, is identified and coagulated. Constant irrigation with warm saline solution with either an endoscope sheath or a common 60-mL syringe helps to maintain the endoscopic view, avoiding surgical delays.

Before entering the sphenoid sinus, a vascularized flap is elevated for eventual closure of the anticipated skull base defect. A nasoseptal pedicled flap with blood supply from the posterior nasal artery, a branch of the sphenopalatine artery, is elevated from the contralateral side. Once elevated, the flap can be stored in the nasopharynx or in the respective maxillary sinus after an antrostomy, thus still providing the surgeon with direct and detailed visualization of the anterior wall of the sphenoid sinus.

Once the flap is secured, a posterior septectomy is performed to allow the 2-nostrils 4-hands technique. Also, ipsilateral posterior ethmoidectomy and wide anterior sphenoidectomy are performed to improve visualization and achieve an adequate working corridor. Septations within the sinus are then flattened.

The next stage of the approach encompasses the lateral aspect of the ventral skull base. This part of the procedure is based on bone removal and drilling to progressively expose the elements of the QS and middle fossa.

An ipsilateral transpterygoid approach is required, which starts with an uncinectomy and enlargement of the maxillary ostium to obtain an antrostomy. In some patients, removal of the bulla ethmoidalis is necessary for a better operative field view. Within the posterior wall of the maxillary sinus, the distal segment of V2 (infraorbital nerve [ION]) and the terminal branches of the maxillary artery are visualized. Removal of this bony wall provides access to these branches and the PPF. The maxillary nerve (V2) is encountered superiorly and laterally in the PPF.

Next, the terminal branches of the maxillary, posterior nasal, and sphenopalatine arteries are dissected and coagulated. The vidian nerve is also identified, and the surrounding bone is drilled down in an anterior to posterior direction. Whenever possible, the vidian nerve and artery, if present, are transposed from the vidian canal and preserved. These measures allow the surgeon to precisely delineate the path of the vidian canal toward the anterior surface of the petrous carotid at its emergence at the foramen lacerum area. Once the vidian nerve is transposed or sectioned, the soft contents of the PPF are lateralized and the base of the pterygoid plate is drilled, completely exposing the sphenoid sinus lateral recess.

The surgeon then focuses toward the medial and inferior limits of the QS. These limits are represented by the horizontal (petrous) and vertical (paraclival) segments of the ICA. At this stage of the approach, the surgeon should be able to visualize the vidian nerve, V2, and ION laterally. The ipsilateral optic canal, paraclinoid ICA, and lateral optic-carotid recess (LOCR) must be identified. The region that is anterior to the ICA siphon at the paraclinoid area and inferior to the LOCR (optic strut) represents the SOF, which is the superior limit of any approach to the middle fossa. The carotid protuberances, which are bony impressions around the ICA paraclival canals, can be easily recognized in well-pneumatized sinuses.

The entire bone covering the medial aspect of the middle fossa should be drilled, tailoring the specific needs of the pathologic condition. The periosteum of the middle fossa is exposed completely, and the gasserian impression, with all 3 trigeminal branches, is visualized underneath (see **Fig. 2**A). Usually there is no need for complete ICA skeletonization, which is only performed when there is direct disease encasement or in cases in which ICA mobilization or proximal control is required.

Finally, the periosteum can be opened accordingly. In general, there are 3 areas that are initially explored: Meckel's cave and anteromedial and anterolateral cavernous sinus triangles (see **Fig. 2**B).

When the disease is posterior, medial, or directly related to the gasserian ganglion, an incision is made at the QS. The periosteal dural layer overlying its anterior surface is opened, and the lesion can be directly accessed. To avoid abducens nerve injury, its neurophysiology should be used before any incision is performed and the opening should not transgress the level of the superior border of V2. The MCF can also be reached through the anteromedial (between SOF/V1 and V2) and anterolateral (between V2 and V3) triangles, which provide direct access to the subarachnoid space at the temporal fossa. Consequently, tumors such as meningiomas can be resected at that level (**Fig. 3**). Schwannomas are restricted to Meckel's cave and are reached after the periosteum is opened at the QS and the lateral meningeal dura is preserved (**Figs. 4** and **5**). These lesions can even be followed into the PF in selected cases (see **Fig. 4**).

Closure of the dural defect is achieved with the inlay positioning of a collagen sponge, when possible, followed by the positioning of the previously elevated nasoseptal flap, which is secured with Surgicel (Ethicon Inc, A Johnson & Johnson Company, Somerville, NJ, USA) followed by fibrin glue or Duraseal (Covidien, Hazelwood, MO, USA). Merocel (Medtronic Xomed, Jacksonville, FL, USA) packing or Foley balloon is used to buttress the reconstruction. Silastic splints (Doyle Splints, Medtronic, Minneapolis, MN, USA) are used against the denuded septum to avoid synechiae. Antibiotics are given until packing is removed.

Complications

Potential serious complications with this approach largely involve injury to the cranial nerves and ICA. Transient sixth nerve palsy and V1 and/or V2 sensory deficit can occasionally occur when dissection is pursued in the upper portion of Meckel's cave. Difficulties with mastication can also take place when V3 or the undersurface of the gasserian ganglion is manipulated or injured. In addition, some degree of neural impairment cannot be avoided while resecting

certain malignant neoplasms, a fact that should be discussed with the patient during the informed consent process.

Major vascular injuries are not expected with this approach. Nevertheless, the risk for such a complication increases in those cases in which there is ICA involvement or entrapment by the neoplastic process or in cases in which ICA dislocation is required for effective disease removal. Even in these cases, low vascular injury rates can be expected if the surgeon follows basic microneurosurgical principles, uses a detailed knowledge of the vascular anatomy, and carefully manipulates the important neurovascular structures as little as absolutely necessary.

In general, cerebrospinal fluid (CSF) leaks were a major source of complications during the early days of endoscopic endonasal skull base surgery. This risk is markedly lower for the MCF approaches because these approaches generally do not create high-flow leaks. The vascularized mucosal reconstruction technique is ideal to cover the skull base defect and exposed ICA, preventing both CSF leak and ICA adventitia desiccation.

POSTERIOR FOSSA

There are several neurosurgical approaches that can be used for resection of tumors in the PF. Lesions located posterior to the brainstem, including those involving the fourth ventricle, are clearly better accessed through posterior approaches. For example, supracerebellar infratentorial approach is adequate for lesions at the quadrigeminal and cerebellomesencephalic cisterns.[17] Similarly, the suboccipital approach is acceptable for lesions in the posteroinferior compartment of the PF, and telovelar dissection provides excellent exposure for the lesions located superiorly inside the fourth ventricle.[18,19]

Similarly, the posterolateral approaches offer a more comfortable surgical corridor for lesions lateral to the brainstem. The retrosigmoid approach is appropriate for lesions in the cerebellomesencephalic and cerebellopontine cisterns.[19] The far lateral approach is adequate for lesions located at the cerebellomedullary cistern.[20,21]

Thus, transcranial approaches still represent the approach of choice for many masses of the PF. Alternatively, the traditional lateral skull base approaches are not ideally suited for lesions located ventral to the brainstem. Before the development of EEAs, ventrally located lesions of the PF were exposed using complex and often morbid procedures such as the transoral approach, the presigmoid approach,[22] anterior and posterior petrosectomies with or without labyrinthectomy,[22,23]

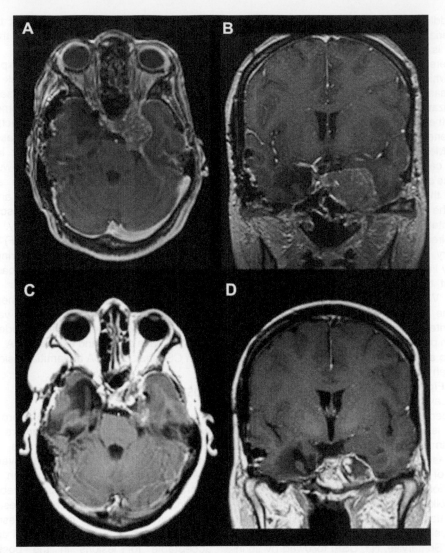

Fig. 3. (*A*) Axial and (*B*) coronal preoperative magnetic resonance images showing a left cavernous sinus tumor in a 34-year-old female patient, consistent with the diagnosis of meningioma. This lesion, which presents a poor hyperintense signal, occupies the entire left cavernous sinus. The lesion extends laterally to the MCF, inferiorly up to the infratemporal fossa, and anteriorly to the orbital apex without invading it. (*C*) Axial and (*D*) coronal postoperative magnetic resonance images after an endoscopic endonasal approach to the middle fossa through the lateral recess of the sphenoid sinus, demonstrating the near total resection with cavernous sinus residual tumor and temporal lobe decompression. On both the preoperative and postoperative images, the right temporal lobe encephalomalacia from a previous craniotomy that was performed elsewhere could be noted.

the extreme lateral approach.[24–26] Often, these approaches provide a limited dissection corridor and force the surgeon to work in the small windows between the cranial nerves, often leading to significant cranial nerve morbidity. Hence, the EEAs provide an ideal alternative to approaching tumors involving the ventral PF, in particular, those with a major component ventral to the brainstem and/or to the lower cranial nerves.[11,14] By using a direct anterior approach, the EEAs allow the surgeon to work in a large window, to work between and not past the cranial nerves, and to devascularize the

tumor early in the case, which is not possible using the lateral approaches.

Indications

To determine whether an EEA is an appropriate choice, it is important to identify the center and extent of the tumor's bony and/or dural attachments. The portion of the tumor to be resected should be ventral to the brainstem and medial to the cranial nerves. For lesions in the intrapeduncular cistern, the tumor should be medial to the third

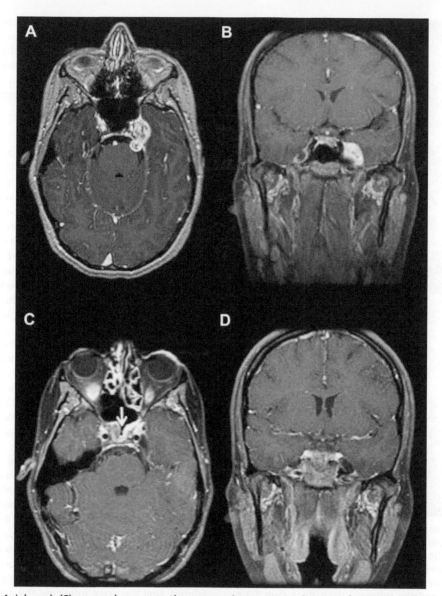

Fig. 4. (*A*) Axial and (*B*) coronal preoperative magnetic resonance images showing a left Meckel's cave schwannoma in a 20-year-old female patient. This lesion, which presents a heterogeneously low to intermediate signal, occupies the inferior cavernous sinus compartment with PF projection. (*C*) Axial and (*D*) coronal postoperative magnetic resonance images after a Meckel's cave endoscopic endonasal approach through the lateral recess of the sphenoid sinus, demonstrating total removal of the lesion.

cranial nerve. For lesions in the prepontine cistern, the tumor should be medial to the sixth cranial nerve. For lesions in the premedullary cistern, the tumor should be medial to the hypoglossal nerves.

The transclival approach can be used for either extradural or intradural lesions of the PF. Chordomas and chondrosarcomas are examples of lesions that can be purely extradural; however, these lesions may often have an intradural component (**Fig. 6**). Alternatively, meningiomas and neurenteric cysts are lesions that mainly occur

intradurally in the PF. Some tumors such as craniopharyngiomas and some pituitary adenomas can also descend from the sellar and suprasellar areas and require an endonasal transclival approach for complete resection.

The main advantage of an endonasal route for appropriate lesions is that in these approaches, the vital structures are located lateral to the tumor and there is no need for neural tissue retraction or dissection in between cranial nerves. Frequently, the nerves and perforating arteries are pushed

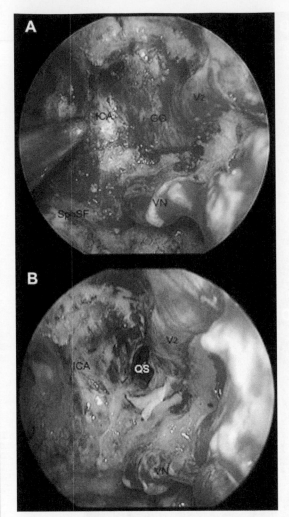

Fig. 5. Intraoperative view of an endoscopic endonasal approach to the MCF for a trigeminal schwannoma. (A) Bone removal in the ventral cranial base with exposure of the gasserian ganglion (GG), ICA, and maxillary nerve (V2). The relation of the vidian nerve (VN) and the sphenoid sinus floor (Sph SF) to the ICA can be observed. (B) Intraoperative view at the end of the tumor resection through the QS.

away by the tumor, which allows direct visualization and safe tumor debulking. Furthermore, these approaches devascularize durally based lesions, such as clival meningiomas, during the tumor exposure, allowing most of the dural origin of these lesions to be resected early in the case and providing a more thorough tumor resection (Fig. 7).

Anatomic Considerations

The clivus can be divided into 3 portions along its rostrocaudal axis (Fig. 8). The upper third includes the dorsum sellae and posterior clinoids down to the level of the sellar floor. The middle third extends from the lower extent of the sella down to the sphenoid floor. The lower third extends from the sphenoid floor to the foramen magnum.

Each third of the clivus has a respective subarachnoid anatomy that can be analyzed in 3 different modules.

Upper third of the clivus

The rostral extension of the superior portion of the clivus is bound by the dorsum sellae in the midline and the posterior clinoids in the paramedian region.

It is important to understand that 2 layers of dura cover the inner side of the sella: the periosteal and the meningeal layers. These layers are found only where there is bone; indeed, the sella has 2 layers in the face, floor, and back wall, between which run the venous channels that communicate both cavernous sinuses, such as the superior, inferior, and posterior intercavernous sinuses (PIS), respectively. The sella has only a single meningeal layer laterally separating it from the cavernous sinus. This concept is important when performing a pituitary transposition, in which the capsule of the gland should not be transgressed and the pituitary ligaments should be detached from the medial cavernous sinus wall. This way, the pituitary gland can be transposed superiorly.

The PIS is located behind the pituitary and is exposed once the gland is elevated. The dorsum sellae is posterior to the PIS. The clival dura harboring the basilar venous plexus is also posterior to the dorsum sellae. Dural opening at that level exposes the interpeduncular cistern guarded laterally by Liliequist membrane and the posterior communicating arteries, the respective perforating arteries, and the third nerves. Posteriorly, the mesencephalon, the basilar bifurcation, the posterior cerebral arteries, and the superior cerebellar arteries limit the area. Inferiorly, the area is bound by the inferior horizontal lamina of Liliequist membrane (Fig. 9A).

Middle third of the clivus

The bony aspect of this region is limited superiorly by the sellar floor and inferiorly by the sphenoid rostrum, which is found at the level of the sphenoid floor in well-pneumatized sphenoid sinuses. Laterally, the ICA paraclival protuberances limit the area. Once the bony structures are removed, the clival dura is exposed with the basilar venous plexus within. It is important to understand that a segment of the sixth cranial nerve's pathway is between the 2 layers of clival dura just before reaching Dorello's canal.

Intradurally, the prepontine cistern is found with the bilateral sixth cranial nerves limiting the space

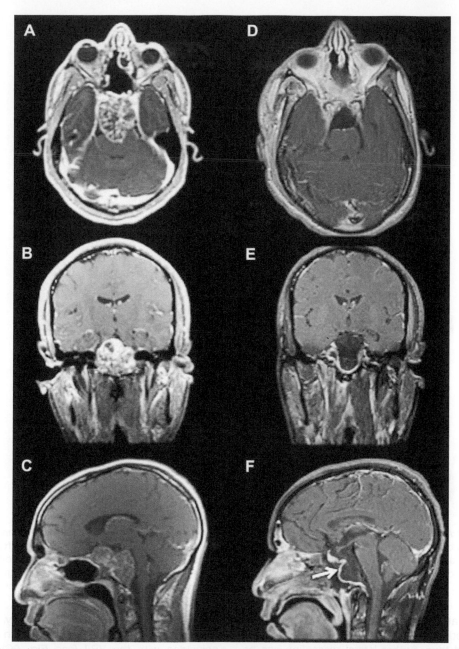

Fig. 6. (A) Axial, (B) coronal, and (C) sagittal preoperative magnetic resonance images showing a large recurrent clival chordoma in a 27-year-old male patient. This heterogeneously hyperintense lesion involves the entire clival area, with posterior dislocation of the pons, lateral extension up to both petrous apexes, and invasion of the cavernous sinuses. (D) Axial, (E) coronal, and (F) sagittal postoperative magnetic resonance images after an endoscopic endonasal approach to the clival area, demonstrating the complete removal of the lesion. The arrow shows the enhancing nasoseptal flap that has been used to reconstruct the skull base defect.

laterally. Posteriorly, the pons is seen with the basilar artery and its branches, including the anteroinferior cerebellar artery (see **Fig. 9**B). The inferior limit of this space is the pontomedullary junction and the vertebrobasilar junction (VBJ).

Inferior third of clivus

The inferior third of the clivus encompasses the anterior aspect of the foramen magnum inferiorly. The superior border is at the sphenoid rostrum junction at the level of the floor of the sphenoid

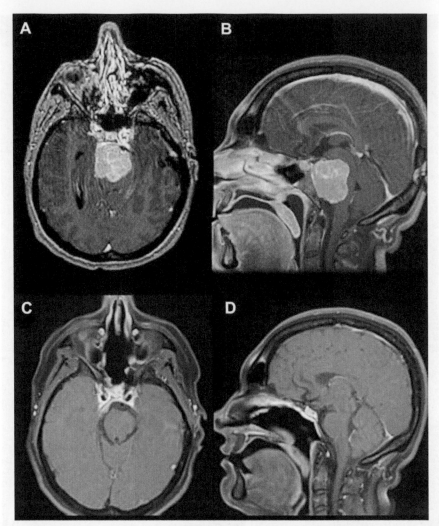

Fig. 7. (*A*) Axial and (*B*) sagittal preoperative post contrast-enhanced T1-weighted magnetic resonance images showing a clival meningioma in a 32-year-old female patient. The lesion appears slightly enhanced after intravenous contrast injection and is located posterior to the clivus mostly on the midline. Dural attachment on the right tentorial edge can also be seen. (*C*) Axial and (*D*) sagittal postoperative magnetic resonance images after an endoscopic endonasal approach to the clival area, demonstrating the complete removal of the lesion.

sinus. Bilaterally, the inferior third of the clivus is not limited directly by the ICA as in the middle third, and thus, further lateral dissection can be safely pursued.

The petroclival synchondrosis is present laterally and can be followed all the way to the jugular foramen. The occipital condyles are positioned in the anterior portion of the foramen magnum and limit the amount of lateral exposure at the inferior part of the clivus. When medial condilectomy is performed to augment the lateral exposure to include the subarachnoid origin of the vertebral artery, the lateral limit is the twelfth cranial nerve traveling inside the hypoglossal canal.

Intradurally, the inferior third of the clivus approaches the premedullary cistern, with the medulla located posteriorly. Superiorly, the limit is at the pontomedullary junction, which generally coincides with the VBJ (see **Fig. 9**C). Consequently, the sixth cranial nerve is not considered at risk at this level. On the other hand, if lateral extension through the condyle is performed, the twelfth cranial nerve limits the approach laterally. If a supracondylar approach is extended through the jugular tubercle, direct exposure of the ninth, tenth, and eleventh cranial nerves is obtained, guarding the cistern laterally.

Surgical Technique

The initial steps of the approach are the same as described for the MCF. However, once the

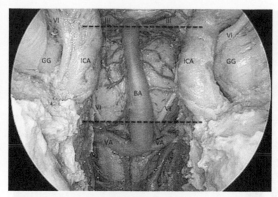

Fig. 8. Panoramic view of a panclivectomy performed on a cadaveric specimen. The boundaries between the upper and middle and the middle and lower thirds of the clivus (*dashed lines*) are visible. BA, basilar artery; GG, gasserian ganglion; VA, vertebral artery; III, oculomotor nerve; VI, abducens nerve.

sphenoid sinus is exposed, a few different steps are necessary to achieve a complete exposure of the clivus, which can be didactically divided into 3 portions based on the clival segments.

Superior third (pituitary transposition/transdorsum sellae)

The surgeon should have a direct view of the sellar protuberance, bilateral ICA impressions, optic canals and optic-carotid recesses, and the clival recess. The bone covering the sellar face is removed to expose the superior intercavernous sinus (SIS), inferior intercavernous sinus (IIS), and the sella-clival junction. Cruciform dural openings are performed above the SIS and on the face of the sella, with care not to transgress the pituitary capsule. After SIS ligation, the dural openings are connected, and the diaphragm is opened all the way to the central aperture to free the pituitary stalk. The ligaments connecting the pituitary capsule to the medial cavernous sinus wall are systematically cut along the lateral contour of the gland. The gland may be mobilized superiorly, enabling exposure of the posterior sellar dura, which is coagulated, and the PIS is transected exposing the dorsum sellae and posterior clinoids.[27] These bony structures are then drilled until eggshell thickness and carefully removed avoiding injury to the ICA and third and sixth cranial nerves. Once these structures have been drilled, the retroclival dura harboring the basilar plexus is visualized. Transgressing the basilar plexus can generate intense venous bleeding, which can be controlled with hemostatic agents such as microfibrillar collagen and absorbable gelatin powder with thrombin.

Intradurally, the dissection follows standard microneurosurgical principles. Tumor debulking should precede extracapsular dissection. Tumors in this location can be firmly attached to the branches of the superior hypophyseal artery, which should be preserved. The basilar apex and perforators are usually pushed posteriorly and attached to tumor capsule. Laterally, the third cranial nerve and the posterior communicating artery with its perforator branches can be densely attached to the capsule and should be dissected carefully (see **Fig. 9**D). Extracapsular dissection should be performed sharply under direct visualization. Craniopharyngiomas can invade the third ventricle, and, consequently, tumor removal can lead the dissection into the ventricle. Care should be taken with the lateral hypothalamic walls and mamillary bodies in these situations. Tumors of the interpeduncular cistern usually push the inferior horizontal lamina of Liliequist membrane downwards, and its preservation helps to decrease subarachnoid blood dissemination to other cisterns.

Middle third (clival recess of sphenoid sinus)

The middle third of the clivus is mostly accessed directly. In well-pneumatized sphenoid sinus, the middle third of the clivus can be a very thin bone forming the deep aspect of the clival recess of the posterior sphenoid sinus. However, rarely the approach is limited to this segment of the clivus, and it is generally combined with the approach for the inferior third of the clivus or with a panclivectomy.

The clival bone is drilled, and the dura and basilar plexus are exposed. Laterally, the approach is limited by the paraclival ICAs, which constrain the approach, particularly in cases in which the disease is located immediately behind the ICA. This is often the case with chordomas and petroclival meningiomas. In such situations, there is a need for further exposure; the ICA canals should be drilled and the periosteum exposed to allow ICA mobilization and better exposure of the anterolateral PF compartment (**Fig. 10**). An important landmark for this exposure is the vidian nerve. The vidian nerve points toward the anterior genu of the ICA, at the level of the foramen lacerum, and helps to identify the petrous ICA in nonpneumatized sphenoid sinuses and/or cases in which the anatomy is deformed by disease. Thus, the ICAs can be mobilized laterally, allowing retrocarotid visualization and dissection.

After meticulous coagulation, the underlying dura is opened at the midline. Neurophysiology and nerve stimulation should be used to identify a sixth cranial nerve that could have been displaced by the tumor. Petroclival

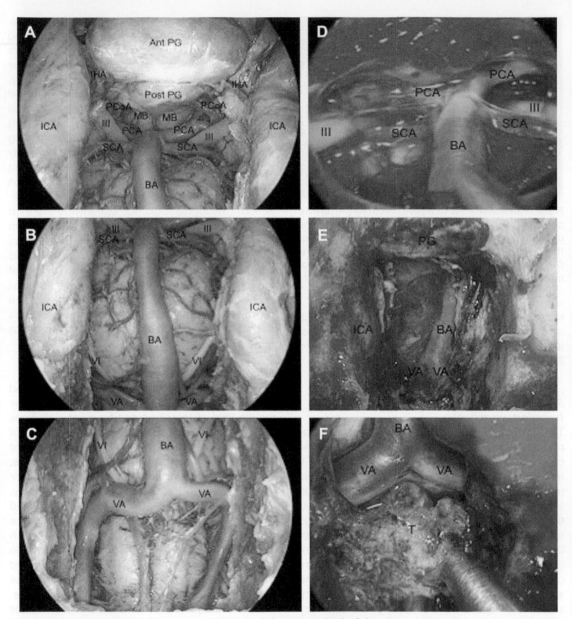

Fig. 9. Cadaveric specimen dissections. (*A*) View of the upper third of the clivus with a 45° endoscope. Ant PG, anterior pituitary gland; BA, basilar artery; IHA, inferior hypophyseal artery; MB, mamillary body; PCA, posterior cerebral artery; PCoA, posterior communicating artery; Post PG, posterior pituitary gland; SCA, superior cerebellar artery; III, oculomotor nerve. (*B*) View of the middle third of the clivus with a 0° endoscope. VA, vertebral artery; VI, abducens nerve. (*C*) View of the lower third of the clivus with a 0° endoscope. Intraoperative views of the endonasal approach to the (*D*) upper third of the clivus, (*E*) middle third of the clivus, and (*F*) lower third of the clivus. T, tumor (meningioma).

meningiomas can displace the sixth cranial nerve medially toward the midline. Image guidance should also be used under computed tomography angiogram visualization to determine the location of the VBJ. Dural opening is performed below the VBJ to assure that the sixth cranial nerve origin at the brainstem remains above.[14]

When performing posterior extracapsular dissection, one must consider the position of the basilar artery and its branches as well as their relationship with the pons (see **Fig. 9E**).

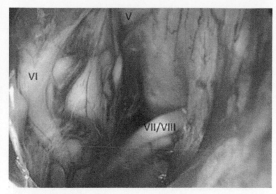

Fig. 10. Lateral view of the brainstem and cranial nerves from a 45° endoscope after resection of a chordoma invading the PF. The left fifth (V) and sixth (VI) cranial nerves as well as the seventh and eighth nerve complex (VII/VIII) are seen.

Inferior third

Initially, the nasal septum is detached from the anterior surface of the sphenoid bone. Extensive mucous removal is necessary for satisfactory exposure of bony landmarks. The basopharyngeal fascia is then stripped from the sphenoid rostrum and clival bone. Next, the sphenoid sinus floor is completely drilled down to the clival dura.

The procedure continues with careful and progressive drilling of the anterior surface of the clivus down to the foramen magnum. Kerrison rongeurs can also be used once the bone has been drilled down to an eggshell thickness. The amount of dural exposure and whether or not the dura itself is opened depends on the nature of the lesion, each approach being tailored to the patient's needs. Because the dura is opened, the medulla is the posterior limit of dissection, and the vertebral arteries must be identified before beginning extracapsular dissection (**Fig. 9F**).

In cases in which there is tumor extension laterally at the level of the lower third of the clivus, further lateral dissection is required. This dissection can conceptually be divided into 3 parts from superior to inferior below the level of the petrous ICA:

1. Infrapetrous (petrous bone below the ICA is removed)
   The area of the foramen lacerum should be exposed, and the dense fibrous tissue connections with eustachian tube should be transected. The infrapetrous bone is drilled under V3 and below the petrous ICA.
2. Supracondylar or transjugular tubercle approach (occipital bone medial to the petroclival synchondrosis and above the occipital condyle is removed)

As the dissection follows the petroclival synchondrosis inferiorly, ninth, tenth, and twelfth cranial nerves should be investigated with neurophysiology monitoring.

3. Transcondylar (medial condylectomy is performed)
   The hypoglossal nerve is the lateral limit; once again neurophysiology monitoring is essential. This lateral extension allows for identification of the proximal aspect of the vertebral artery.

Finally, reconstruction of the cranial defect is achieved with inlay collagen matrix, followed by the pedicled vascularized flap. Occasionally, a foramen magnum exposure cannot be totally covered by the nasoseptal flap. In these situations, reconstruction augmentation is necessary and can be usually obtained with fat graft and/or Alloderm (LifeCell Corp, Woodlands, TX, USA). The reconstruction is then buttressed with Merocel packing or Foley balloon. Silastic splints are used against the denuded septum to avoid synechiae. Antibiotics are given until packing is removed. Rarely, a lumbar drain is placed. However, the lumbar drain is often installed for obese patients, for high flow leaks, and/or in situations with hemorrhage into the subarachnoid space.

Complications

As in the EEA to the MCF, cranial nerves pose a major source of potential complications in EEAs to the PF. Specifically at risk are the third cranial nerve in approaches to the superior third of the clivus, the sixth nerve in approaches to the middle third, and the twelfth cranial nerve in approaches to the inferior third. Meticulous dissection and detailed knowledge of the course of the sixth cranial nerve from the PF to the SOF is mandatory to avoid palsies. Continuous nerve monitoring can be helpful in identifying and avoiding the nerve, especially when dealing with extensive clival deformities caused by tumor growth.

Because the ICA is generously exposed, and even at times manipulated, there is a potential risk for vascular injuries. Once again, anatomic knowledge and a proper surgical technique are the surgeon's best allies to avoid these highly undesirable events.

CSF leaks were a major source of complications during the early days of endoscopic endonasal skull base surgery. Nevertheless, with the introduction and refinement of the pedicled nasoseptal flaps and other vascularized alternative reconstructions,[28–33] the incidence of CSF leaks and postoperation-related morbidity has decreased dramatically, rendering the technique feasible and safe in experienced hands.

REFERENCES

1. Cappabianca P, Alfieri A, de Divitiis E. Endoscopic endonasal transsphenoidal approach to the sella: towards functional endoscopic pituitary surgery (FEPS). Minim Invasive Neurosurg 1998;41:66.
2. Cappabianca P, Alfieri A, Thermes S, et al. Instruments for endoscopic endonasal transsphenoidal surgery. Neurosurgery 1999;45:392.
3. Cappabianca P, Cavallo LM, de Divitiis E. Endoscopic endonasal transsphenoidal surgery. Neurosurgery 2004;55:933.
4. Carrau RL, Jho HD, Ko Y. Transnasal-transsphenoidal endoscopic surgery of the pituitary gland. Laryngoscope 1996;106:914.
5. Jho HD, Carrau RL. Endoscopic endonasal transsphenoidal surgery: experience with 50 patients. J Neurosurg 1997;87:44.
6. Prevedello DM, Doglietto F, Jane JA Jr, et al. History of endoscopic skull base surgery: its evolution and current reality. J Neurosurg 2007;107:206.
7. Cavallo LM, Messina A, Gardner P, et al. Extended endoscopic endonasal approach to the pterygopalatine fossa: anatomical study and clinical considerations. Neurosurg Focus 2005;19:E5.
8. de Divitiis E, Cappabianca P, Cavallo LM, et al. Extended endoscopic transsphenoidal approach for extrasellar craniopharyngiomas. Neurosurgery 2007;61:219.
9. de Divitiis E, Cavallo LM, Esposito F, et al. Extended endoscopic transsphenoidal approach for tuberculum sellae meningiomas. Neurosurgery 2008;62:1192.
10. Kassam A, Snyderman CH, Mintz A, et al. Expanded endonasal approach: the rostrocaudal axis. Part I. Crista galli to the sella turcica. Neurosurg Focus 2005;19:E3.
11. Kassam A, Snyderman CH, Mintz A, et al. Expanded endonasal approach: the rostrocaudal axis. Part II. Posterior clinoids to the foramen magnum. Neurosurg Focus 2005;19:E4.
12. Kassam AB, Prevedello DM, Carrau RL, et al. The front door to Meckel's cave: an antero medial corridor via expanded endoscopic endonasal approach- technical considerations and clinical series. Neurosurgery 2009;64(Suppl 3):71–82 [discussion: 82–3].
13. Prevedello DM, Thomas A, Gardner P, et al. Endoscopic endonasal resection of a synchronous pituitary adenoma and a tuberculum sellae meningioma: technical case report. Neurosurgery 2007; 60:E401 [discussion: E401].
14. Stippler M, Gardner PA, Snyderman CH, et al. Endoscopic endonasal approach for clival chordomas. Neurosurgery 2009;64:268.
15. Gardner PA, Kassam AB, Thomas A, et al. Endoscopic endonasal resection of anterior cranial base meningiomas. Neurosurgery 2008;63:36.
16. Jane JA Jr, Han J, Prevedello DM, et al. Perspectives on endoscopic transsphenoidal surgery. Neurosurg Focus 2005;19:E2.
17. Jittapiromsak P, Little AS, Deshmukh P, et al. Comparative analysis of the retrosigmoid and lateral supracerebellar infratentorial approaches along the lateral surface of the pontomesencephalic junction: a different perspective. Neurosurgery 2008;62: ONS279.
18. Mussi AC, Rhoton AL Jr. Telovelar approach to the fourth ventricle: microsurgical anatomy. J Neurosurg 2000;92:812.
19. Samii M, Gerganov VM. Surgery of extra-axial tumors of the cerebral base. Neurosurgery 2008; 62:1153.
20. Liu JK, Couldwell WT. Far-lateral transcondylar approach: surgical technique and its application in neurenteric cysts of the cervicomedullary junction. Report of two cases. Neurosurg Focus 2005;19:E9.
21. Wen HT, Rhoton AL Jr, Katsuta T, et al. Microsurgical anatomy of the transcondylar, supracondylar, and paracondylar extensions of the far-lateral approach. J Neurosurg 1997;87:555.
22. Al-Mefty O, Ayoubi S, Kadri PA. The petrosal approach for the resection of retrochiasmatic craniopharyngiomas. Neurosurgery 2008;62:ONS331.
23. Chanda A, Nanda A. Partial labyrinthectomy petrous apicectomy approach to the petroclival region: an anatomic and technical study. Neurosurgery 2002; 51:147.
24. Arnold H, Sepehrnia A. Extreme lateral transcondylar approach. J Neurosurg 1995;82:313.
25. Liu JK, Sameshima T, Gottfried ON, et al. The combined transmastoid retro- and infralabyrinthine transjugular transcondylar transtubercular high cervical approach for resection of glomus jugulare tumors. Neurosurgery 2006;59:ONS115.
26. Salas E, Sekhar LN, Ziyal IM, et al. Variations of the extreme-lateral craniocervical approach: anatomical study and clinical analysis of 69 patients. J Neurosurg 1999;90:206.
27. Kassam AB, Prevedello DM, Thomas A, et al. Endoscopic endonasal pituitary transposition for a transdorsum sellae approach to the interpeduncular cistern. Neurosurgery 2008;62:57.
28. Fortes FS, Carrau RL, Snyderman CH, et al. Transpterygoid transposition of a temporoparietal fascia flap: a new method for skull base reconstruction after endoscopic expanded endonasal approaches. Laryngoscope 2007;117:970.

29. Fortes FS, Carrau RL, Snyderman CH, et al. The posterior pedicle inferior turbinate flap: a new vascularized flap for skull base reconstruction. Laryngoscope 2007;117:1329.

30. Oliver CL, Hackman TG, Carrau RL, et al. Palatal flap modifications allow pedicled reconstruction of the skull base. Laryngoscope 2008; 118:2102.

31. Pinheiro-Neto CD, Prevedello DM, Carrau RL, et al. Improving the design of the pedicled nasoseptal flap for skull base reconstruction: a radioanatomic study. Laryngoscope 2007;117:1560.

32. Prevedello DM, Barges-Coll J, Fernandez-Miranda JC, et al. Middle turbinate flap for skull base reconstruction: cadaveric feasibility study. Laryngoscope 2009;119:2094.

33. Zanation AM, Carrau RL, Snyderman CH, et al. Nasoseptal flap reconstruction of high flow intraoperative cerebral spinal fluid leaks during endoscopic skull base surgery. Am J Rhinol Allergy 2009;23:518.

Reconstruction of Dural Defects of the Endonasal Skull Base

Michael E. Sughrue, MD*, Manish K. Aghi, MD, PhD

KEYWORDS

- Draf 3 procedure • Macroadenoma • Foley balloon
- Cribriform

The last decade has seen a marked increase in the ability to remove cranial base lesions with minimal disturbance to the unaffected brain or cranial bone. Improved endoscopic and surgical technology have made intracranial surgery partly or entirely within tight spaces, such as the nasal cavity, obviating a craniotomy or brain retraction to approach lesions of the anterior cranial fossa, sella, clivus, and even many off-midline structures.

Although the possibility of performing complex intracranial procedures without a skin incision or a craniotomy is appealing for many, the limited space makes a neat dural incision and watertight dural closure essentially impossible. While the risk of postoperative cerebrospinal fluid (CSF) leak is manageable in purely intrasellar surgery, because larger lesions are addressed via the endonasal approaches and a greater area of the cranial base is disrupted to expose these lesions, reconstruction of these defects becomes more important, and more difficult.

Several techniques have been used to attempt to repair these defects. Admittedly, no current technique is perfect in all situations; however, existing repair methods represent significant improvements, and are an essential part of the repertoire of anyone contemplating endonasal endoscopic approaches to the cranial base.

BASIC PRINCIPLES OF REPAIR

Perhaps the sole factor working in favor of successful repair of large cranial base defects is the well-vascularized and highly proliferative nasal mucosa surrounding the defect. If allowed to, mucosa overgrows even large defects, providing a lasting barrier against CSF egress via secondary intention. Perhaps the most important tool for repairing these defects is the recognition during the exposure that preservation of as much mucosa as possible with its native blood supply, prevention of unnecessary barriers to mucosal contact with the closure construct, such as unnecessary bony spurs, and minimization of unnecessary mucosa trauma or excessive cauterization probably all improve the likelihood of a permanent mucosa seal being formed.

Another critical feature of successful repair is layered closure. Regardless of closure method, if continued CSF egress is permitted by the method, even if the flow rate is modest, it can maintain and eventually epithelialize a cranionasal fistula, and prevent a permanent mucosal seal from forming at the edges of the defect. Simply put, each additional layer of closure provides one more barrier around which the CSF must go to enter the nose. Although there is a limit, in general, the more layers of different closure materials, the better.

Finally, once the layered closure is in place, it is important to assure that it can resist reasonable stresses without moving. Various different methods for achieving this have been described including the use of bioabsorbable plates to buttress the intradural portion of the repair, the temporary implantation and inflation of the balloon of a Foley catheter, and securing thicker portions of the repair to surrounding tissue using the U-Clip (Medtronic, Minneapolis, MN, USA). Regardless of

Department of Neurological Surgery, University of California at San Francisco, 505 Parnassus Avenue, San Francisco, CA 94117, USA
* Corresponding author.
E-mail address: SughrueM@Neurosurg.UCSF.Edu

Neurosurg Clin N Am 21 (2010) 637–641
doi:10.1016/j.nec.2010.07.004
1042-3680/10/$ — see front matter © 2010 Elsevier Inc. All rights reserved.

the method used, the repair must be given some supporting structure to provide a head start for healing, because extrusion of the repair construct almost guarantees failure.

REPAIR MATERIALS
Nonvascularized Autografts

Autografts are the classic endonasal repair substrates, and can be used to serve several functions in the repair of these defects. Although these are technically simple to harvest and place, they are devascularized tissue, and generally are slowly resorbed and replaced by viable tissue, as opposed to forming their own healthy tissue.

Fat is the most commonly used autograft, and can easily be harvested from the lower abdominal quadrant or the lateral thigh. Fat grafts have come into common use because they are easily malleable and shapeable, and thus not only serve as a barrier to CSF egress but also can prevent the prolapse of neural tissue, like the optic apparatus, through the bony defect left after the approach. Although fat grafts are compressible, there is a limit, and overpacking the defect with fat can cause mass effect and neurologic deficit. The authors have found a variant of the bath-plug technique to be useful in making the fat graft into a firm source of support without the risk of compression-critical structures. In this technique, a slightly oversized piece of fat is wrapped in Surgicel, which is encircled with a 4-0 suture with the ends of the suture threaded through the holes of an absorbable buttressing plate. After introducing the fat into the cavity and tucking the ends of the plate under the edges of the bony defect, the suture is pulled tight against the buttressed plate to compact the fat behind the plate. If sized correctly this fat can form a good seal, and obliterate the potential site of neural prolapsed with minimal risk of overpacking.

Fascia lata can be harvested from the lateral thigh and can be taken at the same time as fat. As a biologic covering, it might be better incorporated into the eventual healed tissue than synthetic grafts. There is a minor risk of injury to lateral femoral cutaneous nerve, so the benefits of fascia should be tempered against this, especially if fat is not going to be used in the repair.

Vascularized Mucosal Flaps

Although harvesting these flaps can be complex and time consuming, their intact blood supply, their large potential surface area, and their thick tissue mass makes them an important recent development in endonasal surgery at the skull base. It is important to plan these flaps into the

exposure if they are to be part of the closure, as not only do most endonasal approaches involve procedures that potentially could injure the blood supply of these flaps, namely the sphenopalatine artery and its branches, but also the flap needs to be safeguarded in some region of the nose that will not be in the primary working axis of the surgery, such as the choana or the maxillary sinus. The ideal location to store the flap depends on the approach, and this should be planned ahead.

Nasoseptal flap

This is a workhorse vascularized mucosal flap, owing to the relative simplicity of elevating this flap with its blood supply, its large potential surface area, and the simplicity by which it can be mobilized to cover defects in nearly every region of the skull base.[1] The flap is based on the posterior nasal branch of the sphenopalatine artery, which is identified by locating the natural osteum of the sphenoid sinus and the choana, between which the artery runs. Using monopolar cautery, the mucosa is incised on the lower edge of the sphenoid osteum and the upper edge of the choana from lateral to medial onto the nasoseptal mucosa. The mucosa incisions spread rostrally and caudally to widen the flap on the nasal septum, but care should be taken not to bring the upper incision too high on the septal mucosa until anterior to the middle turbinate, for fear of injury to the olfactory epithelium. The incisions continue from posterior to anterior, widening to the maximum width possible just anterior to the middle turbinate, stopping at the mucosa-epithelium junction. The flap is then elevated off the nasal septum with a Cottle or other periosteal dissector (**Fig. 1**) and stored in a safe place until needed.

Inferior turbinate flap

The inferior turbinate flap represents a back-up flap when the nasoseptal flap is not an option, usually when previous transphenoidal surgery has either cut or otherwise devascularized the nasoseptal mucosa.[2] This flap is based on the posterolateral nasal artery, a branch of the sphenopalatine artery. Given its early take off after the sphenopalatine foramen, it has a short vascular pedicle in the nasal vault, and thus it is typically necessary to perform a complete uncinectomy, anterior ethmoidectomy, and a wide maxillary antrostomy, to identify and skeletonize the spheno-palatine artery through the posterior maxillary sinus wall following it medially into the nasal vault. The posterolateral nasal artery is then followed onto the inferior turbinate, and a mucosal flap is

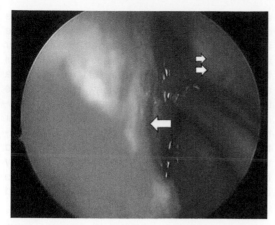

Fig. 1. An intraoperative photo depicting elevation of a nasoseptal mucosal flap. An elevator is used to elevate the flap (*double small arrows*) off the septal bone (*single large arrow*) subperiosteally in an anterior-to-posterior direction.

elevated from the medial surface of the turbinate up to the anterior head of the turbinate.

Tunneled periosteal flaps

In cases when both the nasoseptal and inferior turbinate flaps are not available, it is possible to harvest pericranium through a linear hemicoronal scalp incision.[3] After performing a wide maxillary antrostomy, the sphenopalatine artery is followed out into the pterygopalatine fossa, the vidian nerve is sacrificed, and the pterygopalatine ganglion is mobilized so that the medial pterygoid plate can be drilled to provide room for the flap. The posterolateral maxillary wall is removed in part to communicate the sinus with the infratemporal fossa. After a pericranial graft is harvested based on the anterior branch of the superficial temporal artery, a lateral canthotomy incision is used to dissect the temporalis muscle down the pterygomaxillary fissure and the lateral maxillotomy made internally. After soft tissue dilation of the tract with tracheostomy dilators passed over guidewires, the pericranium is tunneled into the nasal cavity through the maxillary tunnel created endoscopically, and rotated into position.

Alternatively, to close anterior skull base defects, for example after a transcribriform approach, a pericranial flap can be tunneled through the frontal sinus through a small trephination in the nasion. This technique obviously is used following a wide bilateral frontal sinusotomy (ie, Draf 3 procedure).

Rescue flaps

In the rare case when the nasoseptal, inferior turbinate, and tunneled transpterygoid flaps are not available, other more technically challenging flaps

have been described. A somewhat smaller flap from the middle turbinate based on the posterior sphenopalatine branches can be raised with some difficulty.[4] In rare circumstances, the palatal mucosa can be harvested and a flap elevated based on the descending palatine arteries.[5]

Nonautogenous Grafts and RStructural Material

Various materials for providing a barrier to CSF egress are commercially available, most notably bovine pericardium and dural matrix. Few data support the use of one material over another, what is important is that these layers provide a smooth, flat surface for mucosa to grow over, and that they completely cover the defect. The authors have found the use of a single row of a bioabsorbable plate (Stryker) to be a useful buttress to keep the material from leaving the defect under normal physiologic stress.

Biologic Adhesives

A wide variety of adhesive materials exist, with different durations needed for absorption. Although no specific data exist supporting their use, it seems wise to provide a more watertight seal by applying one of these adhesives to the edges of the repair. The authors have been successful with BioGlue (CryoLife, Kennesaw, GA, USA), particularly with repair of small sellar defects, owing to its thick consistency and long duration before it is biologically degraded. No specific data support the use of one material over another at present.

REGION-SPECIFIC CLOSURE ISSUES
Sella

Sellar closure is one of the more straightforward areas to repair for neurosurgeons, largely because of the ability to preserve the arachnoid in most cases, particularly with pituitary adenomas. The intact arachnoid makes this a low-flow CSF (and thus low-risk) case, and as such, with simple repair techniques the authors seldom experience CSF leaks with conventional repair techniques. Also, the lateral bone of the anterior sellar wall provides a good ledge for placing a buttress plate for securing the repair.

Sellar lesions with a fat graft (with macroadenomas >1 cm) are closed by packing the sella and tightening the fat using the bath-plug technique described. A single-row bioabsorbable plate is tucked under the lateral sellar bone. After covering the face of the plate with dural matrix, a bioglue is applied to the edges and face of the repair in 2 stages to provide 2 layers of adhesive.

Tuberculum Sella and Planum Sphenoidale

The tuberculum sella and planum sphenoidale are possibly the most difficult areas of the midline skull base to close effectively and safely through the endonasal approach. The reason for this is largely the presence of the optic nerves in the lateral portion of the repair. Many lesions addressed through the transplanar/transtubercular approaches, most notably craniopharyngiomas, have an above-average risk of CSF leak because of the frequent need to enter into the ventricles during the intradural portion of the procedure. Given the inherent risks of overpacking the defect, or buttressing the repair with a plate tucked behind the bone edges,

a mucosal flap is highly advised when closing these defects, and this should be planned into the approach with these cases. In combined intrasellar and suprasellar pathology, the authors find it useful to maintain some of the dural ring of the diaphragma sella, if allowed by the pathology (such as some large macroadenomas), to repair the 2 regions separately, and to reduce the total area any single layer has to span to cover the defect. Temporary buttressing of the repair with a Foley balloon, inflated under direct endoscopic visualization, is probably the best way to secure the repair until the flap becomes adherent to the underlying bone and implants.

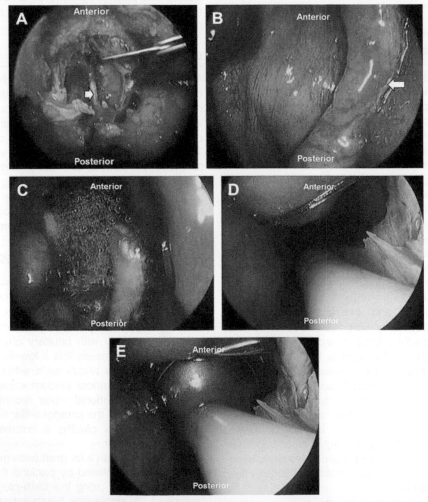

Fig. 2. Repair of a skull base defect after a midline transcribriform approach. The view is looking superiorly using a 0° endoscope. (*A*) The bone and dural defect after removal of the tumor and affected dura. The falx is indicated by the arrow. (*B*) The nasoseptal flap rotated into position and approximated to the edge of the defect; note that the flap is arranged to conform to the contours of the irregular bony defect (*arrow*). (*C*) Dural sealant applied to the edges of the repair. (*D, E*) Foley balloon inflated under direct visualization to buttress the repair.

Cribriform Plate

Although the optic nerve is at less risk with these lesions than with repairs in the tuberculum/planum region, the cribriform region presents unique repair challenges. More specifically, the anterior extent of the defect often is a reach for mucosal flaps based on branches of the sphenopalatine artery. Further, after the frontal sinusotomies, turbinectomies, and anterior septectomy needed to adequately expose cribriform lesions, these defects often are extensive, and it can be difficult to find bone to buttress the layers of the repair. It is probably necessary to brace these repairs with a Foley balloon. The balloon inflation probably helps the flap better conform to the irregular bony cavity that these approaches often create **(Fig. 2)**.

Clivus

Although logistically the clivus is a relatively straightforward region to access and rotate a mucosal flap to reach, these defects often are among the most difficult ones to close effectively. Many times there is nowhere to buttress the defect because of the width of the defect and the lack of gravity counter pressure to keep the graft material taut. Further, the sixth nerve is running in the lateral portion of the defect in many cases, which should be considered when tucking repair material under the bone surfaces. The repair of clival defects in intradural surgery should be planned into the exposure, and bone and dural removal should be minimized as much as allowed by the lesion being addressed.

REFERENCES

1. Hadad G, Bassagasteguy L, Carrau RL, et al. A novel reconstructive technique after endoscopic expanded endonasal approaches: vascular pedicle nasoseptal flap. Laryngoscope 2006;116(10):1882–6.
2. Fortes FS, Carrau RL, Snyderman CH, et al. The posterior pedicle inferior turbinate flap: a new vascularized flap for skull base reconstruction. Laryngoscope 2007;117(8):1329–32.
3. Fortes FS, Carrau RL, Snyderman CH, et al. Transpterygoid transposition of a temporoparietal fascia flap: a new method for skull base reconstruction after endoscopic expanded endonasal approaches. Laryngoscope 2007;117(6):970–6.
4. Prevedello DM, Barges-Coll J, Fernandez-Miranda JC, et al. Middle turbinate flap for skull base reconstruction: cadaveric feasibility study. Laryngoscope 2009;119:2094–8.
5. Oliver CL, Hackman TG, Carrau RL, et al. Palatal flap modifications allow pedicled reconstruction of the skull base. Laryngoscope 2008;118(12):2102–6.

Making the Transition from Microsurgery to Endoscopic Trans-Sphenoidal Pituitary Neurosurgery

Isaac Yang, MD[a], Marilene B. Wang, MD[b],
Marvin Bergsneider, MD[a],*

KEYWORDS

- Microsurgery • Trans-sphenoidal pituitary neurosurgery
- Endoscopic

Endoscopic technology has revolutionized surgical approaches to the paranasal sinuses and the skull base. Initially limited in its scope of applications, the accepted indications for the use of the endoscope to address various disease pathologies is increasingly being adopted and advocated by both skull base surgeons and patients.[1] The evolution of endoscopic trans-sphenoidal pituitary surgery is the natural development and extension of endoscopic technology to the standard microscopic trans-sphenoidal approach to pituitary surgery.[2–7]

While endoscopy provides some inherent advantages in its ability to visualize areas of the sella that are otherwise obscured in the microscopic approach, most neurosurgeons were trained to use the microscope for pituitary surgery, and adoption of endoscopic techniques has been limited to date. There are several potential reasons, including unfamiliarity with the equipment and view. At the authors' institution, a punctuated transition from the traditional, endonasal microscopic technique to the two-surgeon, endonasal endoscopic technique occurred in early 2008. This article reviews the published experience of others plus introduce our insights into the development of an endoscopic pituitary program. While initially challenging, this transition to endoscopic trans-sphenoidal pituitary surgery can yield rewards in the form of superior visualization and potentially more complete tumor resections. The question of whether improved surgical outcomes and reduced complications will materialize will require a comparison of a large series of patients with long-term follow-up.

TRANS-SPHENOIDAL PITUITARY SURGERY

The intimate proximity of the pituitary gland to critical structures in this central location presents unique challenges in the surgical management of pituitary pathology. Victor Horsley is commonly credited with the first successful transcranial surgical management of a pituitary lesion in the late 1800s.[1,7–10] Subsequently, Schloffer is noted to have reported the first trans-sphenoidal approach for tumor removal.[1,7–9,11,12] Cushing introduced the trans-septal trans-sphenoidal procedure in 1910, and in his series reported difficulty with suprasellar extending tumors, poor

[a] UCLA Department of Neurosurgery, David Geffen School of Medicine at UCLA, Box 956901, 10833 Le Conte Avenue, Los Angeles, CA 90095, USA
[b] UCLA Division of Head and Neck Surgery, David Geffen School of Medicine at UCLA, 200 UCLA Medical Plaza, Los Angeles, CA 90095, USA
* Corresponding author.
E-mail address: mbergsneider@mednet.ucla.edu

Neurosurg Clin N Am 21 (2010) 643–651
doi:10.1016/j.nec.2010.07.008
1042-3680/10/$ — see front matter © 2010 Published by Elsevier Inc

illumination, and cerebrospinal fluid (CSF) leakage, which led to the abandonment of this approach by Cushing and his colleagues.[7,8,12–14]

In the late 1950s, Guiot reintroduced this approach with the enhancement of intraoperative fluoroscopy, which permitted an improved ability to guide instruments to the sella and an improved ability to achieve total tumor resection.[7,8,14] Hardy is credited with revolutionizing and re-establishing the trans-sphenoidal approach in the 1960s by combining intraoperative fluoroscopy with the use of the operative microscope.[1,7,9,12,15–18] The introduction of the microscope to pituitary surgery introduced the modern era of trans-sphenoidal surgery, and the wide adoption of the trans-sphenoidal approach to pituitary lesions.[1,9,13,15,17,18] Improving visualization with fluoroscopy and microscopy improved the safety and efficacy of pituitary surgery, which was refined over the subsequent 40 years.[11,12,19–41]

The surgical technique with the microscopic approach is largely limited by the narrow corridor of the nasal speculum. The width of this corridor is a function of the approach, with the purely endonasal approach[42–44] generally necessitating a narrower speculum compared with the traditional sublabial technique. The speculum creates a line-of-sight view of the sella. For intrasellar microadenomas, the surgeon is provided with complete visualization of the entire tumor with some degree of stereoscopic perspective. For larger macroadenomas, however, the field of view can be incomplete.

Because the surgeon may be unable to directly visualize the entire tumor, various blind resection techniques are used. Sweeping motions with various angled pituitary curettes can effectively deliver soft tumor tissue, particularly if aided by a descending diaphragma sella. There are situations, however, in which the probability of an incomplete resection increases. These include a limited sellar bony opening, particularly exacerbated by an incompletely pneumatized sphenoid sinus.[11,12,19–41,45–48] Firm, rubbery tumors can be particularly challenging, especially if adherent to surrounding structures. In general, invasive tumors within the cavernous sinus have been considered off limits with the speculum-based, microscopic approach.

ENDOSCOPIC TRANS-SPHENOIDAL PITUITARY SURGERY

Over the past decade, with the improvements in digital video, optics, light sources, and video monitors, endoscopic trans-sphenoidal pituitary surgery has emerged as an important innovation in pituitary surgery.[13,49–51] To some, the endoscope is simply an alternative visualization device used instead of the microscope. In many cases, surgeons have opted to use the endoscope in lieu of the microscope, performing the operation in essentially an identical manner. Although angled-lens endoscopes may offer some added value to visualize residual tumor, a smaller sellar opening and exposure is a common limiting factor. In some cases, a hybrid endoscopic-assisted approach is used, essentially augmenting the view, but not the approach, to the sella. Some of the published series of endoscopic pituitary surgery use this limited approach. Whereas the surgical endoscope is an alternative visualization device relative to the microscope, its use allows a virtually completely different surgical approach for larger tumors.

> Trans-sphenoidal endoscopic approaches range from:
> Endoscopic-assisted surgery using a speculum;
> Single-surgeon single-nostril endoscopy with limited sellar opening
> Single-surgeon, single or dual nostril endoscopy with expanded exposure
> Dual-surgeon, dual nostril expanded approach (so-called expanded, endoscopic endonasal approach, or EEEA[52,53]).

The authors adopted EEEA at their institution in early 2008.

The EEEA is a fundamentally different surgical approach compared with the traditional speculum-based transnasal trans-sphenoidal. In the authors' experience, the removal of a pituitary tumor is more akin to removing a convexity meningioma. It is based on several key concepts. First is wide (expanded) exposure of the entire extent of the tumor involvement. For example, tumor involvement of the anterior cranial fossa requires removal of the tuberculum sella and possibly the planum sphenoidale, whereas wide exposure of the dura over the cavernous sinus is required for tumors involving that compartment. To do so, extensive drilling of the sphenoid sinus is often required, so much so that this technique is more invasive than other so-called minimally invasive techniques. Just as blind dissection is generally unacceptable with open craniotomy approaches to tumors, the same philosophy is applied to pituitary and other parasellar tumors.

A second concept relates to using routine microsurgical techniques, including bimanual manipulation and dissection of neurovascular structures and tumor tissue under direct visualization. The binostril approach allows more degrees of freedom compared with uninostril and endonasal speculum-based approaches. In addition, the endoscope allows the use of standard microsurgical instruments, including the Rhoton microdissectors (Codman, Raynham, MA, USA) and ultrasonic aspirators.

To maintain constant visualization of the area of dissection, the authors use the dual-surgeon technique (**Fig. 1**). One surgeon holds the endoscope, constantly moving the endoscope to maintain the surgical field centered, as well as avoiding conflict with the instruments used by the surgeon removing the tumor. By using various angled endoscopes, areas not visualized by other approaches can be safely accessed.[4–6,9,54–57] This improved visualization may enhance the identification of critical neurovascular structures, which may reduce the complications of pituitary surgery and may improve tumor resection by identifying residual tumor in the sella.[4–6,9,12,13,55,56,58–73] Endoscopic transsphenoidal pituitary surgery also may reduce blood loss and improve operating time for difficult pituitary procedures.[3–6,60,74] This may be due to the reduced injury to the nasal and septal mucosa, which may result in less bleeding.[74] Hence, endoscopic trans-sphenoidal pituitary surgery may allow for access to the sella more quickly and smoothly, and provide enhanced visualization, particularly of the region near the sella turcica.[3,55,73,74] Endoscopic trans-sphenoidal pituitary surgery also may reduce hospital stay, improve patient satisfaction, and decrease the need for postoperative nasal packing.[2,7]

The expanded exposure does impose added complexity with regard to reconstruction, particularly with patients with intraoperative CSF leaks. With small sellar openings, it is generally easier

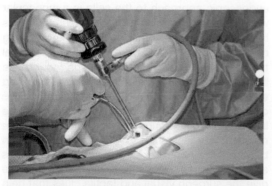

Fig. 1. The dual-surgeon technique maintains constant visualization of the area of dissection, as one surgeon holds the endoscope, constantly moving the endoscope to maintain the surgical field centered and avoiding conflict with the instruments used by the surgeon removing the tumor.

to support and buttress fat grafts. The wide drilling of the skull base with EEEA surgeries can be extensive, and therefore it may not be possible to secure bone grafts (or other substitutes) to buttress the fat (or other material) grafts. This had led to the wide use of vascularized, nasoseptal flaps for reconstruction.[75–81]

Finally, a rarely mentioned challenge with the use of endoscopes is the fact that blood, running down the endoscope shaft, can intermittently obscure the view. This requires frequent irrigation of the endoscope with saline. For surgeons accustomed to the continuous view afforded by the speculum and surgical microscope, this can be unnerving. For experienced endoscopic surgeons, this is not a serious issue. This issue should not be confused with the ability to control surgical bleeding. Although one might assume that surgical bleeding would be problematic using the endoscope, it is the authors' experience that it is far easier to control and stop bleeding with the use of the dual-surgeon, endoscopic approach. The authors routinely enter the cavernous sinus using this technique; this area is actually much harder to control using a speculum and microscope due to the fact it is not generally in the surgical field of view.

Making the Transition from the Microscope to the Endoscope

An early study by Stankiewicz initially suggested a steep learning curve to endoscopic surgery with a higher complication rate for less experienced surgeons.[82] His experience suggests a learning curve of approximately 90 cases.[83–85] Other studies also suggest a similar number for the learning curve for standardization of this novel approach and for gaining ease and familiarity with endoscopic trans-sphenoidal surgery.[63,64]

More recently, Sonnenburg and colleagues[1] reported their series of the first 45 minimally invasive pituitary cases done at the University of North Carolina by both otolaryngology and neurosurgery in joint cases. In their series, they reported an overall CSF leak rate of approximately 4% and suggested that there is not a steep learning curve to minimally invasive pituitary surgery with the collaboration between otolaryngology and neurosurgery at an academic medical center. In another retrospective analysis of the otolaryngology experience for the endoscopic trans-sphenoidal learning curve, Marks also suggested that the learning curve is not steep and that significant advancement on this curve can be achieved during residency training.[86,87] Other recent reports additionally have suggested that the learning curve to endoscopic surgery is not a steep one and that significant advancement on this curve can occur during a rigorous residency training program.[86,88,89]

Kabil and colleagues[8] reported on their retrospective analysis of endoscopic and transseptal approaches to pituitary surgery. In their experience, they suggested that the enhanced visualization of the endoscope improves the ability to differentiate normal pituitary from tumor tissue and also permits exceptional visualization of the suprasellar and parasellar regions of pituitary tumor extension. Their series of 300 endoscopic trans-sphenoidal pituitary surgeries reported a CSF leak of less than 2% with improvement as the surgeon advances along the learning curve. Furthermore, their large retrospective analysis suggested that it may be possible to improve tumor resection and reduce complication rates using the enhanced visualization of endoscopy to trans-sphenoidal pituitary surgery.[8] Another recent report by Jarrahy and colleagues[13] in a small series of consecutive patients also suggested that tumor fragments that can only be identified endoscopically may be present in over one-third of pituitary tumor cases. In a recent large cohort, Cappabianca and colleagues[63] reported their postoperative complications in a series of 146 consecutive cases of endoscopic trans-sphenoidal surgery for pituitary adenomas. Their CSF leak rate was only 2%, and their morbidity and mortality rate was comparable to modern microscopic trans-sphenoidal results.[90]

A recent systematic review of the reported literature on endoscopic trans-sphenoidal pituitary surgery indicates that over 800 patients have now been treated with endoscopic trans-sphenoidal approaches with little morbidity and even less mortality.[9] The overall rate of CSF leak was 6% (the most common complication), and the mortality rate was 0.2% in this data analysis. This large analysis of a pooled cohort of patients suggests that endoscopic trans-sphenoidal pituitary surgery can be performed safely with minimal complications and almost no mortality. In comparison to traditionally reported results from trans-sphenoidal surgery, this meta-analysis suggests that endoscopic trans-sphenoidal surgery is similar in effectiveness and risk as traditional approaches to pituitary surgery.[2,7,9,11,12,21,37,40,90,91] It has been suggested that outcomes with endoscopic trans-sphenoidal pituitary surgery may improve as it becomes widely adopted and neurosurgeons advance along the learning curve and aggregate cumulative experience over time.[9] Among limitations of the literature reporting on endoscopic trans-sphenoidal pituitary surgery are the limited

long-term results, as this approach has only been widely employed for the past decade.

Over the past 2 years, the authors have successfully made the transition from microscopic to fully endoscopic pituitary surgery at their institution, having performed over 180 operations in this time. The authors' ability to adopt this approach was facilitated by the fact that both surgeons (MB, MBW) were already adept and highly experienced with endoscopic operations.[92–103] As such, there was virtually no learning curve with respect to the use of an endoscope.

What was required in the authors' case was formal training in the EEEA technique, which they acquired over an intense 4-day hands-on course. Understanding the unique surgical anatomy, surgical techniques, and teamwork training were key to the authors' successful transition. In the authors' opinion, it is not a procedure that should be casually adopted. It requires a dedicated team, including surgical nurses and ancillary personnel familiar with the equipment and procedure.

For their team, the authors incorporated an experienced rhinologic surgeon (MBW) in these cases. Although not necessary for the surgical approach for many routine cases, the rhinologic surgeon can be invaluable for complex or repeat operations. Because the seamless dual-surgeon teamwork is most important for these difficult cases, the authors use the dual-surgeon technique for all cases. Preoperative discussion of the sinonasal sequelae of the surgery by the rhinologic surgeon is also helpful in preparing patients for expectations during the recovery period. Furthermore, they can provide the optimal postoperative care with outpatient endoscopic nasal lavages and surveillance.

One of the suggested disadvantages of the endoscopic approach to the sella is a monocular view instead of the binocular view neurosurgeons have become accustomed to, particularly among neurosurgeons who have received minimal training in the use of the endoscope.[1,2,63] These limitations, however, are mitigated with improving endoscope technologies, significantly larger high-definition visualization video screens, and the increasing incorporation of endoscopic training in neurosurgery residencies.[1,13] Dynamic interaction between the left- and right-handed instruments and coordinated movement of the endoscope give the surgeon visual and tactile clues that help to compensate for the monocular view. The authors have found that a significantly large (50 in or greater size) high-definition screen (**Fig. 2**) can be immersive in its visualization, and can mitigate many of the problems caused by the

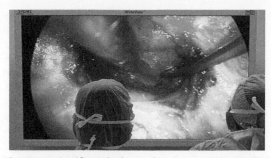

Fig. 2. A significantly large (50 in or greater size) high-definition (HD) flat panel screen can be immersive in its visualization and may mitigate many of the problems caused by the monocular view provided by the endoscope.

monocular view provided by the endoscope. The extra space that endoscopic videos and monitors used to take now can be minimized by flat screen high definition visualization technology. Furthermore, digital imaging improvements with dual chips at the tip of the endoscope may permit three-dimensional visualization with technological advancement.[104] Lastly, as the value of endoscopic techniques becomes more apparent, the use of the endoscope during residency training may also improve, and eventually begin to incorporate virtual reality surgery training similar to what pilots use for virtual reality flight simulators in their training.[1,104]

FUTURE APPLICATIONS OF ENDOSCOPIC TRANS-SPHENOIDAL PITUITARY SURGERY

With increasing cumulative experience with the endoscopic trans-sphenoidal technique for pituitary surgery, the improved visualization and less steep learning curve will facilitate more widespread acceptance of endoscopic pituitary surgery as a valid alternative to the trans-septal trans-sphenoidal microscopic approach to pituitary tumors. If not a complete alternative, endoscopic assisted pituitary surgery will also become more widespread as endoscopy can easily supplement standard microscopic approaches to pituitary tumors. As transnasal endoscopic approaches to the skull base are increasingly refined in technology and skill, additional applications of this technology may permit skull base approaches through the planum sphenoidale and tuberculum sellae for the removal of giant suprasellar macroadenomas, which may otherwise require an open craniotomy for surgical management.[59] This extended endoscopic trans-sphenoidal approach to the skull base may expand the applications of endoscopy technology

to skull base surgery.[51,87,105−107] Furthermore, robotic enhancement of endoscopic trans-sphenoidal pituitary surgery may be possible as thoracic and abdominal robotic surgery systems are miniaturized for application in endonasal endoscopic surgery.[49,50] Lastly, integration of improved optical aids and operating instruments as well as constantly improving neuronavigation may also improve the ease with which endoscopic trans-sphenoidal pituitary surgery can be learned.

Future studies should focus on technique refinement, increasing standardization, and the adoption of novel extensions and applications of this technology. The collaboration between otolaryngologists and neurosurgeons is important for further developing successful endoscopic trans-sphenoidal pituitary surgery and improving care for patients.[61−63] Objective evidence is needed to validate whether the improved visualization results in superior patient outcomes and reduced clinical complications, and if this novel technique can be reasonably taught in a controlled, supervised setting in residency training programs. Additional outcomes data are needed to evaluate long-term outcomes and define the boundaries of endoscopic trans-sphenoidal pituitary surgery.

REFERENCES

1. Sonnenburg RE, White D, Ewend MG, et al. The learning curve in minimally invasive pituitary surgery. Am J Rhinol 2004;18(4):259−63.
2. Nasseri SS, McCaffrey TV, Kasperbauer JL, et al. A combined, minimally invasive transnasal approach to the sella turcica. Am J Rhinol 1998; 12(6):409−16.
3. Cho DY, Liau WR. Comparison of endonasal endoscopic surgery and sublabial microsurgery for prolactinomas. Surg Neurol 2002;58(6):371−5 [discussion: 375−6].
4. Jho HD. Endoscopic transsphenoidal surgery. J Neurooncol 2001;54(2):187−95.
5. Jho HD, Alfieri A. Endoscopic endonasal pituitary surgery: evolution of surgical technique and equipment in 150 operations. Minim Invasive Neurosurg 2001;44(1):1−12.
6. Alfieri A, Jho HD. Endoscopic endonasal cavernous sinus surgery: an anatomic study. Neurosurgery 2001;48(4):827−36 [discussion: 836−7].
7. Sonnenburg RE, White D, Ewend MG, et al. Sellar reconstruction: is it necessary? Am J Rhinol 2003; 17(6):343−6.
8. Kabil MS, Eby JB, Shahinian HK. Fully endoscopic endonasal vs transseptal transsphenoidal pituitary surgery. Minim Invasive Neurosurg 2005;48(6): 348−54.

9. Tabaee A, Anand VK, Barron Y, et al. Endoscopic pituitary surgery: a systematic review and meta-analysis. J Neurosurg 2009;111(3):545–54.

10. Horsley V. Disease of the pituitary gland. Br Med J 1906;1:323.

11. Dew LA, Haller JR, Major S. Transnasal trans-sphenoidal hypophysectomy: choice of approach for the otolaryngologist. Otolaryngol Head Neck Surg 1999;120(6):824–7.

12. Ciric I, Ragin A, Baumgartner C, et al. Complications of trans-sphenoidal surgery: results of a national survey, review of the literature, and personal experience. Neurosurgery 1997;40(2):225–36 [discussion: 236–7].

13. Jarrahy R, Berci G, Shahinian HK. Assessment of the efficacy of endoscopy in pituitary adenoma resection. Arch Otolaryngol Head Neck Surg 2000;126(12):1487–90.

14. Welbourn RB. The evolution of transsphenoidal pituitary microsurgery. Surgery 1986;100(6):1185–90.

15. Hardy J, Wigser SM. Trans-sphenoidal surgery of pituitary fossa tumors with televised radiofluoroscopic control. J Neurosurg 1965;23(6):612–9.

16. Hardy J. Transphenoidal microsurgery of the normal and pathological pituitary. Clin Neurosurg 1969;16:185–217.

17. Hardy J. Excision of pituitary adenomas by trans-sphenoidal approach. Union Med Can 1962;91:933–45.

18. Hardy J, Vezina JL. Transsphenoidal neurosurgery of intracranial neoplasm. Adv Neurol 1976;15:261–73.

19. Ross DA, Wilson CB. Results of transsphenoidal microsurgery for growth hormone-secreting pituitary adenoma in a series of 214 patients. J Neurosurg 1988;68(6):854–67.

20. Jane JA Jr, Laws ER Jr. The surgical management of pituitary adenomas in a series of 3093 patients. J Am Coll Surg 2001;193(6):651–9.

21. Barker FG 2nd, Klibanski A, Swearingen B. Trans-sphenoidal surgery for pituitary tumors in the United States, 1996–2000: mortality, morbidity, and the effects of hospital and surgeon volume. J Clin Endocrinol Metab 2003;88(10):4709–19.

22. Ciric I, Mikhael M, Stafford T, et al. Trans-sphenoidal microsurgery of pituitary macroadenomas with long-term follow-up results. J Neurosurg 1983;59(3):395–401.

23. Charpentier G, de Plunkett T, Jedynak P, et al. Surgical treatment of prolactinomas. Short- and long-term results, prognostic factors. Horm Res 1985;22(3):222–7.

24. Chandler WF, Schteingart DE, Lloyd RV, et al. Surgical treatment of Cushing's disease. J Neurosurg 1987;66(2):204–12.

25. Maira G, Anile C, De Marinis L, et al. Prolactin-secreting adenomas: surgical results and long-term follow-up. Neurosurgery 1989;24(5):736–43.

26. Mampalam TJ, Tyrrell JB, Wilson CB. Trans-sphenoidal microsurgery for Cushing disease. A report of 216 cases. Ann Intern Med 1988;109(6):487–93.

27. Tyrrell JB, Lamborn KR, Hannegan LT, et al. Transsphenoidal microsurgical therapy of prolactinomas: initial outcomes and long-term results. Neurosurgery 1999;44(2):254–61 [discussion: 261–3].

28. Guidetti B, Fraioli B, Cantore GP. Results of surgical management of 319 pituitary adenomas. Acta Neurochir (Wien) 1987;85:117–24.

29. Fahlbusch R, Buchfelder M. Present status of neurosurgery in the treatment of prolactinomas. Neurosurg Rev 1985;8:195–205.

30. Fahlbusch R, Buchfelder M, Muller OA. Transsphenoidal surgery for Cushing's disease. J R Soc Med 1986;79(5):262–9.

31. Yang SY, Zhu T, Zhang JN, et al. Trans-sphenoidal microsurgical management of pituitary adenomas. Microsurgery 1994;15(11):754–9.

32. Guilhaume B, Bertagna X, Thomsen M, et al. Transsphenoidal pituitary surgery for the treatment of Cushing's disease: results in 64 patients and long-term follow-up studies. J Clin Endocrinol Metab 1988;66(5):1056–64.

33. Boggan JE, Tyrrell JB, Wilson CB. Trans-sphenoidal microsurgical management of Cushing's disease. Report of 100 cases. J Neurosurg 1983;59(2):195–200.

34. Davis DH, Laws ER Jr, Ilstrup DM, et al. Results of surgical treatment for growth hormone-secreting pituitary adenomas. J Neurosurg 1993;79(1):70–5.

35. Hammer GD, Tyrrell JB, Lamborn KR, et al. Transsphenoidal microsurgery for Cushing's disease: initial outcome and long-term results. J Clin Endocrinol Metab 2004;89(12):6348–57.

36. Abosch A, Tyrrell JB, Lamborn KR, et al. Transsphenoidal microsurgery for growth hormone-secreting pituitary adenomas: initial outcome and long-term results. J Clin Endocrinol Metab 1998;83(10):3411–8.

37. Black PM, Zervas NT, Candia GL. Incidence and management of complications of trans-sphenoidal operation for pituitary adenomas. Neurosurgery 1987;20(6):920–4.

38. Tindall GT, Oyesiku NM, Watts NB, et al. Transsphenoidal adenomectomy for growth hormone-secreting pituitary adenomas in acromegaly: outcome analysis and determinants of failure. J Neurosurg 1993;78(2):205–15.

39. Tindall GT, Herring CJ, Clark RV, et al. Cushing's disease: results of trans-sphenoidal microsurgery with emphasis on surgical failures. J Neurosurg 1990;72(3):363–9.

40. Semple PL, Laws ER Jr. Complications in a contemporary series of patients who underwent trans-sphenoidal surgery for Cushing's disease. J Neurosurg 1999;91(2):175–9.

41. Ebersold MJ, Quast LM, Laws ER Jr, et al. Long-term results in trans-sphenoidal removal of nonfunctioning pituitary adenomas. J Neurosurg 1986;64(5):713–9.

42. Fatemi N, Dusick JR, de Paiva Neto MA, et al. The endonasal microscopic approach for pituitary adenomas and other parasellar tumors: a 10-year experience. Neurosurgery 2008;63:244–56 [discussion: 256].

43. Dusick JR, Fatemi N, Mattozo C, et al. Pituitary function after endonasal surgery for nonadenomatous parasellar tumors: Rathke's cleft cysts, craniopharyngiomas, and meningiomas. Surg Neurol 2008;70(5):482–90 [discussion: 490–1].

44. Fatemi N, Dusick JR, Gorgulho AA, et al. Endonasal microscopic removal of clival chordomas. Surg Neurol 2008;69(4):331–8.

45. Abe T, Ludecke DK. Recent primary transnasal surgical outcomes associated with intraoperative growth hormone measurement in acromegaly. Clin Endocrinol (Oxf) 1999;50(1):27–35.

46. Abe T, Ludecke DK. Recent results of secondary transnasal surgery for residual or recurring acromegaly. Neurosurgery 1998;42(5):1013–21 [discussion: 1021–2].

47. Abe T, Ludecke DK. Recent results of primary transnasal surgery for infradiaphragmatic craniopharyngioma. Neurosurg Focus 1997;3(6):e4.

48. Abe T, Ludecke DK. Transnasal surgery for prolactin-secreting pituitary adenomas in childhood and adolescence. Surg Neurol 2002;57(6):369–78 [discussion: 378–9].

49. O'Malley BW Jr, Weinstein GS. Robotic skull base surgery: preclinical investigations to human clinical application. Arch Otolaryngol Head Neck Surg 2007;133(12):1215–9.

50. Hanna EY, Holsinger C, DeMonte F, et al. Robotic endoscopic surgery of the skull base: a novel surgical approach. Arch Otolaryngol Head Neck Surg 2007;133(12):1209–14.

51. Lee SC, Senior BA. Endoscopic skull base surgery. Clin Exp Otorhinolaryngol 2008;1(2):53–62.

52. Kassam AB, Gardner PA, Snyderman CH, et al. Expanded endonasal approach, a fully endoscopic transnasal approach for the resection of midline suprasellar craniopharyngiomas: a new classification based on the infundibulum. J Neurosurg 2008;108(4):715–28.

53. Kassam A, Thomas AJ, Snyderman C, et al. Fully endoscopic expanded endonasal approach treating skull base lesions in pediatric patients. J Neurosurg 2007;106(Suppl 2):75–86.

54. Jankowski R, Auque J, Simon C, et al. Endoscopic pituitary tumor surgery. Laryngoscope 1992;102(2):198–202.

55. Cappabianca P, Cavallo LM, de Divitiis E. Endoscopic endonasal trans-sphenoidal surgery. Neurosurgery 2004;55(4):933–40 [discussion 940–1].

56. Gamea A, Fathi M, el-Guindy A. The use of the rigid endoscope in trans-sphenoidal pituitary surgery. J Laryngol Otol 1994;108(1):19–22.

57. Sethi DS, Pillay PK. Endoscopic management of lesions of the sella turcica. J Laryngol Otol 1995;109(10):956–62.

58. Helal MZ. Combined microendoscopic trans-sphenoid excisions of pituitary macroadenomas. Eur Arch Otorhinolaryngol 1995;252(3):186–9.

59. Schwartz TH, Stieg PE, Anand VK. Endoscopic trans-sphenoidal pituitary surgery with intraoperative magnetic resonance imaging. Neurosurgery 2006;58(Suppl 1):ONS44–51 [discussion: ONS44–51].

60. White DR, Sonnenburg RE, Ewend MG, et al. Safety of minimally invasive pituitary surgery (MIPS) compared with a traditional approach. Laryngoscope 2004;114(11):1945–8.

61. Cappabianca P, Alfieri A, Colao A, et al. Endoscopic endonasal trans-sphenoidal approach: an additional reason in support of surgery in the management of pituitary lesions. Skull Base Surg 1999;9(2):109–17.

62. Cappabianca P, Alfieri A, Colao A, et al. Endoscopic endonasal trans-sphenoidal surgery in recurrent and residual pituitary adenomas: technical note. Minim Invasive Neurosurg 2000;43(1):38–43.

63. Cappabianca P, Cavallo LM, Colao A, et al. Surgical complications associated with the endoscopic endonasal trans-sphenoidal approach for pituitary adenomas. J Neurosurg 2002;97(2):293–8.

64. Cappabianca P, Cavallo LM, de Divitiis E. Collagen sponge repair of small cerebrospinal fluid leaks obviates tissue grafts and cerebrospinal fluid diversion after pituitary surgery. Neurosurgery 2002;50(5):1173–4 [author reply 1174].

65. Jho HD, Carrau RL, Ko Y, et al. Endoscopic pituitary surgery: an early experience. Surg Neurol 1997;47(3):213–22 [discussion 222–3].

66. Esposito F, Cappabianca P, Del Basso De Caro M, et al. Endoscopic endonasal trans-sphenoidal removal of an intra-suprasellar schwannoma mimicking a pituitary adenoma. Minim Invasive Neurosurg 2004;47(4):230–4.

67. Cavallo LM, Briganti F, Cappabianca P, et al. Hemorrhagic vascular complications of endoscopic trans-sphenoidal surgery. Minim Invasive Neurosurg 2004;47(3):145–50.

68. Cappabianca P, Cavallo LM, Valente V, et al. Sellar repair with fibrin sealant and collagen fleece after endoscopic endonasal trans-sphenoidal surgery. Surg Neurol 2004;62(3):227–33 [discussion 233].

69. Cappabianca P, Cavallo LM, Esposito F, et al. Endoscopic endonasal trans-sphenoidal surgery: procedure, endoscopic equipment, and instrumentation. Childs Nerv Syst 2004;20:796–801.

70. Carrau RL, Jho HD, Ko Y. Transnasal–trans-sphenoidal endoscopic surgery of the pituitary gland. Laryngoscope 1996;106(7):914–8.

71. Jho HD, Carrau RL. Endoscopy assisted trans-sphenoidal surgery for pituitary adenoma. Technical note. Acta Neurochir (Wien) 1996;138(12):1416–25.

72. Heilman CB, Shucart WA, Rebeiz EE. Endoscopic sphenoidotomy approach to the sella. Neurosurgery 1997;41(3):602–7.

73. Sethi DS, Stanley RE, Pillay PK. Endoscopic anatomy of the sphenoid sinus and sella turcica. J Laryngol Otol 1995;109(10):951–5.

74. Ogawa T, Matsumoto K, Nakashima T, et al. Hypophysis surgery with or without endoscopy. Auris Nasus Larynx 2001;28(2):143–9.

75. Caicedo-Granados E, Carrau R, Snyderman CH, et al. Reverse rotation flap for reconstruction of donor site after vascular pedicled nasoseptal flap in skull base surgery. Laryngoscope 2010;120(8):1550–2.

76. Nyquist GG, Anand VK, Singh A, et al. Janus flap: bilateral nasoseptal flaps for anterior skull base reconstruction. Otolaryngol Head Neck Surg 2010;142(3):327–31.

77. Zanation AM, Carrau RL, Snyderman CH, et al. Nasoseptal flap reconstruction of high flow intraoperative cerebral spinal fluid leaks during endoscopic skull base surgery. Am J Rhinol Allergy 2009;23(5):518–21.

78. Kang MD, Escott E, Thomas AJ, et al. The MR imaging appearance of the vascular pedicle nasoseptal flap. AJNR Am J Neuroradiol 2009;30(4):781–6.

79. Kassam AB, Thomas A, Carrau RL, et al. Endoscopic reconstruction of the cranial base using a pedicled nasoseptal flap. Neurosurgery 2008;63(Suppl 1):ONS44–52 [discussion ONS52–3].

80. Pinheiro-Neto CD, Prevedello DM, Carrau RL, et al. Improving the design of the pedicled nasoseptal flap for skull base reconstruction: a radioanatomic study. Laryngoscope 2007;117(9):1560–9.

81. Hadad G, Bassagasteguy L, Carrau L, et al. A novel reconstructive technique after endoscopic expanded endonasal approaches: vascular pedicle nasoseptal flap. Laryngoscope 2006;116(10):1882–6.

82. Stankiewicz JA. Complications of endoscopic intranasal ethmoidectomy. Laryngoscope 1987;97(11):1270–3.

83. Stankiewicz JA. Complications of endoscopic sinus surgery. Otolaryngol Clin North Am 1989;22(4):749–58.

84. Stankiewicz JA. Complications in endoscopic intranasal ethmoidectomy: an update. Laryngoscope 1989;99:686–90.

85. Stankiewicz JA. The endoscopic approach to the sphenoid sinus. Laryngoscope 1989;99(2):218–21.

86. Marks SC. Learning curve in endoscopic sinus surgery. Otolaryngol Head Neck Surg 1999;120(2):215–8.

87. Kuppersmith RB, Alford EL, Patrinely JR, et al. Combined transconjunctival/intranasal endoscopic approach to the optic canal in traumatic optic neuropathy. Laryngoscope 1997;107(3):311–5.

88. Kinsella JB, Calhoun KH, Bradfield JJ, et al. Complications of endoscopic sinus surgery in a residency training program. Laryngoscope 1995;105(10):1029–32.

89. Vleming M, Middelweerd RJ, de Vries N. Complications of endoscopic sinus surgery. Arch Otolaryngol Head Neck Surg 1992;118(6):617–23.

90. Laufer I, Anand VN, Schwartz TH. Endoscopic, endonasal extended trans-sphenoidal, transplanum transtuberculum approach for resection of suprasellar lesions. J Neurosurg 2007;106(3):400–6.

91. Carrau RL, Kassam AB, Snyderman CH. Pituitary surgery. Otolaryngol Clin North Am 2001;34(6):1143–55.

92. Bergsneider M. Endoscopic removal of cysticercal cysts within the fourth ventricle: technique and results. Neurosurg Focus 1999;6(4):e8.

93. Bergsneider M. Endoscopic removal of cysticercal cysts within the fourth ventricle. Technical note. J Neurosurg 1999;91(2):340–5.

94. Bergsneider M. Complete microsurgical resection of colloid cysts with a dual-port endoscopic technique. Neurosurgery 2007;60:ONS33–42 [discussion ONS42–3].

95. Bergsneider M, Holly LT, Lee JH, et al. Endoscopic management of cysticercal cysts within the lateral and third ventricles. Neurosurg Focus 1999;6(4):e7.

96. Bergsneider M, Holly LT, Lee JH, et al. Endoscopic management of cysticercal cysts within the lateral and third ventricles. J Neurosurg 2000;92(1):14–23.

97. Dusick JR, McArthur DL, Bergsneider M. Success and complication rates of endoscopic third ventriculostomy for adult hydrocephalus: a series of 108 patients. Surg Neurol 2008;69(1):5–15.

98. Frazee JG, King WA, De Salles AA, et al. Endoscopic-assisted clipping of cerebral aneurysms. J Stroke Cerebrovasc Dis 1997;6(4):240–1.

99. Gravori T, Steineke T, Bergsneider M. Endoscopic removal of cisternal neurocysticercal cysts. Technical note. Neurosurg Focus 2002;12(6):e7.

100. Joo D, Chhetri DK, Wang MB. Endoscopic removal of juvenile nasopharyngeal angiofibromas: a video presentation. Laryngoscope 2008;118(6):e1–3.

101. King WA, Ullman JS, Frazee JG, et al. Endoscopic resection of colloid cysts: surgical considerations using the rigid endoscope. Neurosurgery 1999; 44(5):1103–9 [discussion 1109–11].

102. Sung A, Bergsneider M, Wang MB. Transnasal endoscopic surgery of the cavernous sinus for tissue diagnosis. Laryngoscope 2010;120(2):282–4.

103. Upchurch K, Raifu M, Bergsneider M. Endoscope-assisted placement of a multiperforated shunt catheter into the fourth ventricle via a frontal transventricular approach. Neurosurg Focus 2007;22(4):E8.

104. Levy ML, Nguyen A, Aryan H, et al. Robotic virtual endoscopy: development of a multidirectional rigid endoscope. Neurosurgery 2006;59(Suppl 1): ONS134–41 [discussion ONS134–41].

105. Jho HD. The expanding role of endoscopy in skull-base surgery. Indications and instruments. Clin Neurosurg 2001;48:287–305.

106. Casler JD, Doolittle AM, Mair EA. Endoscopic surgery of the anterior skull base. Laryngoscope 2005;115(1):16–24.

107. Li KK, Teknos TN, Lai A, et al. Traumatic optic neuropathy: result in 45 consecutive surgically treated patients. Otolaryngol Head Neck Surg 1999;120(1):5–11.

Minimally Invasive Neurosurgery for Cerebrospinal Fluid Disorders

Daniel J. Guillaume, MD, MSc

KEYWORDS

- Cerebrospinal fluid • Neuroendoscopy • Hydrocephalus
- Endoscopic third ventriculostomy

The general goals for treating disorders of cerebrospinal fluid (CSF) circulation are restoration of the balance between CSF production and clearance, and elimination of pressure gradients between CSF compartments. In most cases, this translates to fluid diversion via membrane fenestration or shunting. The first implantable shunt valve, invented by Nulsen and Spitz[1] in the 1950s, revolutionized the treatment of hydrocephalus, a previously devastating disease. Unfortunately, despite attempts to make shunt dynamics more physiologic, complications related to shunting have continued to plague patients with hydrocephalus. Advances in shunt technology have failed to improve outcomes or circumvent shunt complications.

As technology continues to modify techniques used to treat neurosurgical conditions, there has been a trend toward techniques that achieve minimal invasiveness with access and visualization provided through the smallest opening possible, with greatest action limited to the point of interest, thus minimizing retraction of normal brain tissue. Advances in minimally invasive neurosurgical techniques, including endoscopy and frameless image guidance, have been part of a major driving force toward development of a superior means to achieve CSF diversion. Paralleling this has been innovation and evolution in the training, experience, knowledge sharing, and familiarity with the endoscope by both practicing neurosurgeons and residents. Applications are rapidly growing and this has had a dramatic effect on the treatment of nearly all disorders of CSF circulation.

This article focuses on minimally invasive approaches to address disorders of CSF circulation. The endoscope has played the major role in changing the way many of these disorders are treated. If studied carefully, these new approaches may also help us better understand the nature of some of these complex dynamic physiologic disorders. To date, the most prevalent use of the endoscope in neurosurgery has been in removing obstructions of CSF flow and/or diverting flow, with little disruption of normal brain tissue. As such, neuroendoscopy has gained most attention in the treatment of focally obstructive entities such as aqueductal stenosis, tumoral hydrocephalus, isolated ventricles, arachnoid cysts, multiloculated hydrocephalus, and fourth ventricular outlet obstructions. Investigative work has also been done using some endoscopic techniques in CSF disorders thought not to be obstructive in nature, including normal pressure hydrocephalus, and hydrocephalus secondary to hemorrhage or infection. The endoscope can also play a key role in treating these disorders by other means, including choroid plexus coagulation, endoscopic shunt placement, and endoscopic assistance of open techniques for CSF diversion.

Using minimally invasive techniques, in many cases shunts can be avoided or removed and craniotomies can be circumvented. For many

Department of Neurosurgery, Oregon Health & Science University, 3303 South West Bond Avenue, Mail Code CH8N, Portland, OR 97239, USA
E-mail address: guillaum@ohsu.edu

Neurosurg Clin N Am 21 (2010) 653–672
doi:10.1016/j.nec.2010.07.005

patients this may translate to less pain, shorter hospital stays, and most importantly, improved outcome. The emphasis of investigations to come will need to focus on outcomes, and statistical evaluations to prove superiority of endoscopic procedures over traditional shunting operations.

DISORDERS OF CSF CIRCULATION AMENABLE TO MINIMALLY INVASIVE NEUROSURGERY

Disorders of CSF circulation most amenable to endoscopic treatment are those that are caused by an identifiable, focal obstruction. **Table 1** lists some conditions that are often successfully treated using endoscopy. In general, obstructions causing disruption of normal CSF flow result in dilatation of the ventricular system proximal to the obstruction, often resulting in compression of brain structures, raised intracranial pressure (ICP), and associated symptoms. Shunting the dilated fluid space has previously treated many of these conditions. Unfortunately, in addition to typical problems that accompany shunting, including infection, misplaced catheter, and malfunction, shunting an isolated fluid space creates a pressure differential across the membranous obstruction that is not physiologic. Endoscopic techniques, on the other hand, can effectively

and more physiologically treat most cases of CSF obstruction by either membrane fenestration or removal of mass lesion, which can result in restoration of normal CSF flow or creation of a bypass into the ventricles or subarachnoid spaces distal to the obstruction.

The classic obstructive condition most commonly treated successfully by endoscopic means is aqueductal stenosis (**Fig. 1**A). Other lesions obstructing CSF flow include: fourth ventricular outlet obstruction (including Chiari Malformation), isolated lateral ventricle due to foramen of Monro stenosis (see **Fig. 1**B), tumors that block CSF flow (see **Fig. 1**C), multiloculated hydrocephalus (see **Fig. 1**D), isolated fourth ventricle due to both aqueductal obstruction and fourth ventricular outlet obstruction (commonly from adhesions) (see **Fig. 1**E), and arachnoid cysts (see **Fig. 1**F). Other conditions that have been investigated as possibly amenable to endoscopic treatment are those classically considered to be forms of communicating hydrocephalus, including hydrocephalus secondary to subarachnoid hemorrhage, normal pressure hydrocephalus, or hydrocephalus secondary to infection. Results with endoscopic treatments of these conditions have been varied and these mixed results are likely to due to an unclear (and possibly heterogeneous) etiology

Table 1
Common disorders of CSF circulation amenable to minimally invasive neurosurgical treatment

Condition	Point of Obstruction	Treatments
Aqueductal stenosis	Cerebral aqueduct	1. Endoscopic third ventriculostomy 2. Aqueductoplasty 3. Removal of mass lesion 4. Endoscopic lamina terminalis fenestration
Isolated lateral ventricle	Foramen of Monro	1. Septum pellucidotomy 2. Foraminoplasty 3. Removal of mass lesion
Isolated fourth ventricle	Cerebral aqueduct and fourth ventricular outlet	1. Aqueductoplasty + lysis of fourth ventricular outlet adhesions 2. Lysis of fourth ventricular adhesions + endoscopic third ventriculostomy 3. Removal of mass lesion
Fourth ventricular outlet obstruction (Chiari)	Fourth ventricular outlet	1. Endoscopic third ventriculostomy 2. Removal of mass lesion
Multiloculated hydrocephalus	Intraventricular adhesions	1. Adhesion lysis
Arachnoid cyst	Multiple locations	1. Cyst fenestration

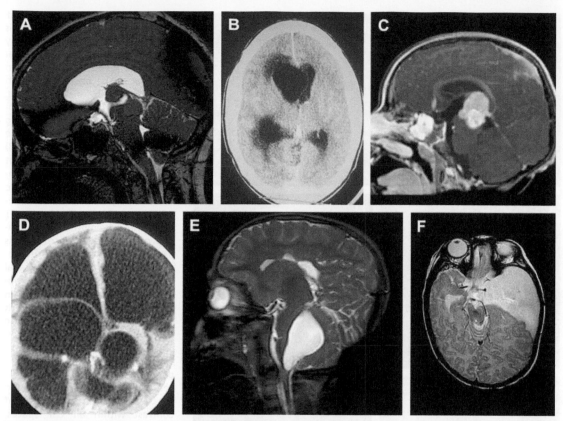

Fig. 1. Disorders of CSF circulation amenable to endoscopic treatment. Disorders most responsive to endoscopic treatment are those that are caused by an identifiable obstruction. Aqueductal stenosis (*A*) leads to dilatation of the third and fourth ventricles with a relatively normal-sized fourth ventricle. Isolated lateral ventricle (*B*), caused by blockage at the level of the foramen of Monro, leads to dilatation of one lateral ventricle with a normal or compressed contralateral lateral ventricle. Tumors involving the pineal region (*C*), posterior third ventricle, or posterior fossa lead to triventricular hydrocephalus, similar to aqueductal stenosis. In multiloculated hydrocephalus (*D*), the presence of multiple intraventricular membranes can lead to expansion of multiple isolated fluid spaces, causing compression of surrounding structures. Isolated fourth ventricle (*E*) can cause dilatation of all 4 ventricles, but will not respond to diversion of only supra- or infratentorial CSF spaces because of lack of communication. Arachnoid cysts (*F*) can directly compress brain structures and may also lead to obstruction of CSF pathways.

behind the mechanism and pathway of CSF flow in these conditions.

APPROACH TO WORKUP OF CSF DISORDER

In general, endoscopic membrane fenestration is most likely to be successful if a clinically significant membranous obstruction can be clearly demonstrated on preoperative imaging. Often, the nature of the obstruction will be obvious on simple preoperative imaging studies such as computed tomography (CT) scan because of significant ventricular dilatation proximal to an obstruction, with normal-sized or compressed ventricles distal. This view has been most commonly demonstrated

in the case of aqueductal stenosis, with dilatation of the lateral and third ventricles in conjunction with a relatively normal-sized fourth ventricle and small-convexity subarachnoid spaces (**Fig. 2**A). Other forms of obstructive hydrocephalus easily diagnosed using only CT include isolated lateral ventricle (see **Fig. 1**B) and isolated fourth ventricle (see **Fig. 1**E). Although CT can demonstrate gross dilatation of isolated fluid spaces relative to normal spaces, in some cases it will be necessary to more closely define the nature of the obstruction, either functionally or anatomically. The 3 imaging studies most useful in this regard are: (1) high-resolution magnetic resonance imaging (MRI) using a constructive interference in the steady-state

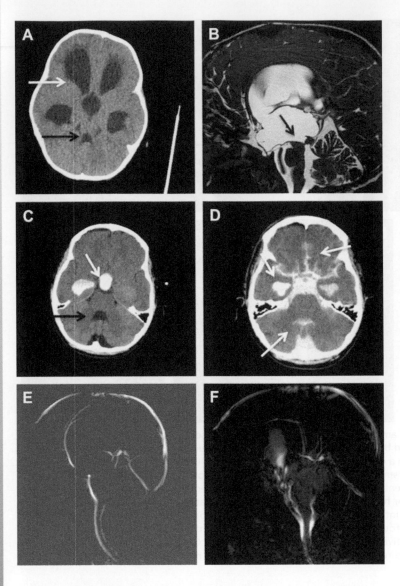

Fig. 2. Imaging workup of CSF disorders. In aqueductal stenosis (A), a head computed tomography (CT) scan shows significant lateral and third ventricular dilatation proximal to the obstruction, with a normal-sized fourth ventricle. High-resolution magnetic resonance imaging (MRI) using a constructive interference in the steady-state (CISS) sequence (B) produces an image with excellent CSF-to-brain contrast demonstrating the branches of the basilar artery and abnormal aqueductal membrane. Head CT following intraventricular instillation of iodinated contrast, in this patient with obstructive hydrocephalus due to aqueductal stenosis (C), demonstrates entrapment of contrast material within lateral and third ventricles with no contrast within fourth ventricle or subarachnoid CSF spaces. Following endoscopic third ventriculostomy (ETV) in the same patient, head CT following intraventricular injection of iodinated contrast shows presence of contrast within all CSF spaces, including the prepontine cistern and subarachnoid space (D). Before ETV, cine phase contrast MRI showed absence of flow in the aqueduct (E). Following ETV (F), the cine sequence shows flow through the third ventricular floor, indicating ventriculostomy patency.

(CISS) sequence, (2) contrast ventriculography, and (3) cine MRI.

MRI scans are performed to localize an obstruction and to provide detailed information needed for surgical planning. In some cases, the planning MRI can be performed at the same time as a scan to be used for frameless stereotactic neuronavigation. Routine T1- and T2-weighted images are obtained in the axial, coronal, and sagittal planes. In addition, a CISS sequence can be performed to identify thin membranes that might interfere with CSF circulation (see **Fig.** 2B). CISS uses fast imaging with steady-state free precession to compensate for slow flow, thereby enhancing the cisternographic effect,[2] producing an image with excellent CSF-to-brain contrast. CISS can be especially useful in imaging the floor of the third ventricle and the contents of the prepontine cistern when

contemplating endoscopic third ventriculostomy (ETV), because Liliequist's membrane, the branches of the basilar artery, and abnormal intraventricular or intracisternal membranes can be visualized (see **Fig.** 2B).

In patients harboring an external ventricular drain placed after removal of infected shunt, or to control acute hydrocephalus, there is an opportunity to evaluate for the presence of functional obstructions by contrast ventriculography. Iodinated contrast (approximately 3 mL), can be carefully instilled into the ventricular catheter after removing an identical quantity of CSF; this is followed by instillation of enough CSF or preservative-free normal saline to flush the contrast agent from the ventricular drain into the ventricular system. The drain is then clamped and ICP is transduced. The patient typically undergoes a head CT immediately following instillation of ventricular contrast, 1 hour later, and in some cases several hours later if there is interest in documenting slow CSF transit. This method is an ideal means to evaluate true functional ventricular obstructions. In some ways it is superior to MRI, as membranes may be observed on high-resolution CISS sequences that may still allow flow due to partial autofenestration not easily interpreted on MRI. Contrast ventriculography will demonstrate entrapment of contrast material within the ventricles proximal to the obstruction (see **Fig. 2**C) or presence of contrast within all CSF spaces including prepontine cistern, and subarachnoid space in the setting of communication of CSF spaces (see **Fig. 2**D). In cases of relative stenosis or narrowing of CSF passageways, a delayed scan may demonstrate eventual progression of contrast to distal CSF spaces, which is often seen in the setting of multiple arachnoid adhesions that have developed after either infection or hemorrhage. The obvious disadvantage of this invasive technique over MRI is that it requires access to CSF spaces.

Because most disorders of CSF circulation are caused by an anomaly in the dynamics of CSF flow, measurements of CSF flow are ideal for diagnosis of CSF flow disorders and also for monitoring in follow-up. Two MRI techniques can reliably measure flow: (1) a cine phase contrast (PC) sequence in which the flow is coded on a gray scale, and (2) a cine phase contrast flow (PCF) sequence in which the velocity is coded on a gray scale but also on a quantitative scale.[3] Velocity measurement is possible by means of flow analysis, with the time parameter given by a signal synchronized on the heartbeat. Cine PC and PCF are now routinely used to assess obstructions in the normal CSF pathways, and also to evaluate patency following treatments (see **Fig. 2**E, F). In obstructive hydrocephalus, cine PC MRI can objectively assess the absence of flow in a given structure such as the aqueduct or foramen of Monro (see **Fig. 2**E, F). Following treatment such as ETV, the cine PCF sequence allows measurement of the flow through the third ventricular floor (see **Fig. 2**E, F).

GENERAL APPROACH TO ENDOSCOPIC MANAGEMENT OF CSF DISORDERS

When it has been determined that a condition is amenable to endoscopic treatment, careful preparation can increase the chance of success and decrease complication rate. This aim usually requires careful study of preoperative imaging, thoughtful evaluation of treatment options, and consideration of the need for frameless neuronavigation.

When planning membrane fenestration, the overall objective is to restore normal CSF balance by creating openings in obstructive membranes that will remain patent, while avoiding trauma to functional brain tissue and/or blood vessels. A straight line from the entry point should traverse the membrane(s) that require fenestration. In many cases, a prior burr hole can be used. At other times, use of multiple burr holes is necessary to adequately and safely fenestrate the important obstructive membranes. The fenestrations should be as large as possible, and there should be as many as possible. Frameless navigation, with stereotactic tracking of the endoscopic tip, can be very useful because disorientation is a frequent encumbrance.

The repertoire of endoscopic equipment for management of complex disorders of CSF circulation should include rigid and in some cases flexible endoscopes, with high-resolution video camera systems, irrigation method, and ability for navigational tracking of the endoscope. The endoscope collection often includes a rigid rod-lens endoscope with good optical quality, variations of viewing angles (typically 0° and 30°), and easy handling. Various mechanical instruments of different sizes such as scissors, grabbers, hooks, puncture needles, biopsy and grasping forceps, bipolar and unipolar coagulation instruments, and Fogarty balloon catheters are useful for safely creating fenestrations.

General techniques for endoscopic approaches have been described.[4–8] In general, endoscopic techniques are performed under general anesthesia. The patient's head rests on a horseshoe headrest or 3-pin fixation when frameless navigation is used. The entry point is determined with the goal of approaching the target with a straight approach, to avoid injury to important structures between the entry point and target (such as the fornix). Side-to-side movement of the endoscope should be avoided. Proper entry can sometimes be accomplished by drawing a line on the preoperative MRI, or the frameless navigation station, from the target through a safe channel (such as the foramen of Monro) and extending this to cross the calvarium. The intersection with the calvarial surface and skin is the entry point for burr hole and incision, respectively. In addition to avoiding important neural structures, care is taken to avoid important vascular structures such as major arterial branches and venous sinuses.

The incision can be linear, but in general should be curvilinear if there is a chance a shunt may be required if the endoscopic procedure fails. A burr hole is created that is large enough to accommodate the working sheath of the endoscope (in some cases up to 1 cm in diameter). A funnel-shaped burr hole, with the narrow portion near the outer skull table, allows endoscopic movement while minimizing the outer defect. After opening the dura, a ventricular needle is inserted into the ventricle initially, if using a free-hand technique, to safely find the ventricle. Some describe placing the operating sheath directly into the ventricle after dural opening; however, the author finds it is safer to first cannulate the ventricle using a smaller diameter ventricular needle. If using image guidance, the operating sheath/trocar can be directly inserted into the ventricle using navigation while tracking the tip of the sheath/trocar. In the case of small or slit-like ventricles, or in cases with distorted anatomy, image guidance improves safety. Image guidance is also beneficial for determination of the ideal entry point and navigation toward target membranes.

Once the endoscope is inserted, the anatomy is inspected to confirm correct location using anatomic landmarks and, if using navigation, this is correlated to landmarks on the workstation. The author does not use continuous irrigation. Instead, lactated Ringer solution is used to flush through the irrigation ports of the endoscope using a hand-held syringe technique only as needed for visualization. This method offers the advantage of tactile feedback regarding ICP. If significant backpressure is encountered, this may indicate a problem with CSF egress, which must be addressed to avoid increases in ICP. One can also leave an external ventricular drain in place during the procedure for continuous measurement of ICP.

Several techniques are available for the management of unexpected bleeding. Small hemorrhages usually cease spontaneously after a few minutes of waiting, or with irrigation. If this fails, a bipolar diathermy probe can be used to achieve hemostasis while using irrigation to improve visualization of the bleeding point. Other techniques include tamponade either with the scope itself, or by placing a small cottonoid down the working sheath and holding pressure using a grabbing instrument. In extreme circumstances, air can be injected into the ventricular system to replace CSF, to transform the ventricular space from liquid to air medium; this aids visualization of bleeding. CSF should not be removed using suction because this can lead to ventricular collapse, potential extra-axial hemorrhage, and worsening of visualization. In extreme circumstances, though very rare, the endoscope can be removed and the operation converted to an open procedure for hematoma evacuation.

SPECIFIC ENDOSCOPIC TECHNIQUES
Endoscopic Third Ventriculostomy

ETV has gained nearly worldwide acceptance as a safe and effective treatment for many causes of pediatric and adult hydrocephalus. Despite the increasing use of this technique, no clear guidelines are available and controversy continues over which patients are appropriate candidates for the procedure. This controversy largely exists due to an overabundance of retrospective case series suggesting relative safety and efficacy of endoscopic procedures over more traditional CSF diversion procedures, and a lack of well-designed prospective randomized trials comparing ETV with shunting.

There is a consensus that ETV is generally indicated as a treatment for any type of hydrocephalus that is caused by obstruction proximal to the fourth ventricular outlet.[9-14] A typical example is shown in **Fig. 3**. ETV has also been successful in the management of CSF obstructions distal to the fourth ventricle, such as Dandy-Walker malformation and Chiari malformations.[15-21]

By studying outcomes, indications for ETV have become more precisely defined.[4,22-38] One of the most controversial issues has been the age at which ETV is likely to be effective. Most reports support that improved outcome after ETV is associated with older age.[12,39-41] Different studies have shown improved outcome in older patients with the cut-off in different studies varying from older than 6 months of age,[11] older than 12 months,[42] and older than 2 years.[12] A few studies, on the other hand, suggest that outcome is not dependent on age.[43,44]

The Canadian Pediatric Neurosurgery Study Group conducted a collaborative study to address the important determinants of outcome after ETV, including age, by pooling 368 patients who underwent ETV from 9 Canadian centers.[45] By multivariate analysis, only age had a significant effect on outcome, with younger patients failing at higher rates, particularly neonates and infants, leading to the conclusion in this study that the only statistically significant variable influencing outcome is age.

Despite this result, some believe that ETV may be a reasonable method of initial CSF diversion in children even younger than 6 months.[46] In a study of 14 patients younger than 6 months with obstructive hydrocephalus treated with ETV, success was obtained in 8 patients (57%). It could be reasoned that ETV should be recommended because it gives an opportunity for shunt independence in a significant proportion of patients, potentially avoiding the long-term complications

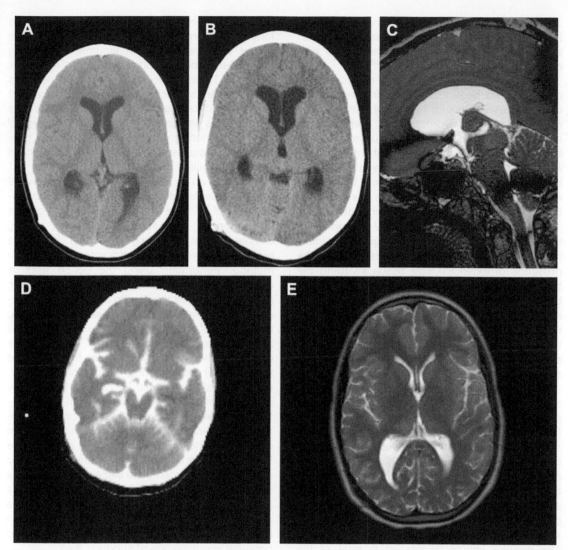

Fig. 3. Case example: ETV with removal of malfunctioning ventriculoperitoneal shunt. This 12-year-old girl was shunted at birth for triventricular hydrocephalus. She presented 1 month after proximal revision with headache, nausea, vomiting, decreased level of consciousness, and bradycardia. Head CT on presentation after removal of 20 mL CSF from shunt reservoir (*B*) showed enlarged lateral and third ventricles compared with baseline scan (*A*). High-resolution sagittal MRI CISS sequence (*C*) showed evidence of obstruction at the level of the aqueduct, and suggested she would be a good candidate for ETV. After ETV, an external ventricular drain was placed and transduced ICPs were normal. Instillation of ventricular iodinated contrast showed communication of all CSF spaces (*D*). MRI scan obtained 3 months later (*E*), when she was feeling "better than baseline," showed ventricles that were smaller than prior well baseline, suggesting partial obstruction or nonideal valve pressure on her original shunt.

associated with a shunt. Conversely, it can be argued that it is equally reasonable to initially shunt these patients, reserving ETV for consideration in the face of a shunt malfunction occurring when older than 2 years.

Outcome is also strongly related to the etiology of hydrocephalus, with success of ETV being ideally suited to those with primary and secondary aqueductal stenosis.[8,22,23,28,31,33,37–39,41,47–77] In

the best candidates, the distal CSF pathways are patent and the basal cisterns are free from adhesions that occur after bleeding or infection. MRI sequences, as described earlier, can delineate the nature of the obstruction. Downward bulging of the third ventricular floor into the prepontine cistern, dilatation of the suprapineal recess into the quadrigeminal cistern, flattening of the mesencephalon, funneling of the upper part of the aqueduct, and normal or even small size of the fourth ventricle are all frequently associated with aqueductal stenosis, and are rarely found with communicating hydrocephalus.[78–80]

In addition to obstructive types of hydrocephalus, ETV has been investigated in the study of communicating types of hydrocephalus, such as normal pressure hydrocephalus, with mixed results.[26,81] Some studies document clinical improvement in up to 70% of patients.[26,29,81,82] Although the mechanism of improvement cannot be explained by the bulk CSF flow theory, the mechanism may become clear in the future as CSF hydrodynamics become better understood.

Relative contraindications to ETV include structural anomalies, such as a very large massa intermedia, a thickened third ventricular floor, or the presence of extensive scar tissue involving the third ventricular floor, prepontine cistern, and basilar artery apex. Other anatomic variations, such as a very narrow third ventricle, an effaced interpeduncular cistern, or slit ventricles, are not in themselves contraindications, but require experience and sometimes frameless navigation for safety and success.[36]

Variations on this technique have been extensively described.[8,22,26,30,31,59,64,71,80,83–86] The patient lies supine with head in slight flexion (approximately 15°) with the head positioned on a horseshoe headrest. If stereotactic guidance is required, as in the case of extremely small ventricles or abnormal anatomy, the head is fixed in a 3-pin headrest. Some frameless navigational systems, which use electromagnetic guidance, can avoid placement of pins, and this can be extremely beneficial in the case of small infants. The monitor should be placed in front of the surgeon to allow the surgeon to operate in a neutral position. A frontal curvilinear incision is preferred over a straight incision to prepare for the possibility of ETV failure and need for shunt placement. The burr hole is typically made approximately 3 cm lateral and 1 cm anterior to the coronal suture, which should always be identified before drilling. These coordinates are based on retrospectively obtained imaging data from 27 patients undergoing ETV.[87] A ventricular needle is first inserted into the right lateral ventricle. Following its removal, the endoscope can be navigated along the path directly into the ventricular system. One should avoid attempting to find the ventricle using the endoscope, even in the case of markedly dilated ventricles, as devastating vascular and neurologic complications can occur. If frameless stereotactic navigation is used, the tip of the endoscope/trocar can be tracked as it enters the ventricular system. Once in the right lateral ventricle, the endoscope is navigated through the foramen of Monro into the third ventricle. The floor of the third ventricle with landmarks including mammillary bodies and infundibular recess is identified. The location of the fenestration depends on the patient's specific anatomy. The placement should avoid damage to the basilar artery and its branches, as well as the infundibulum. The typical location is made in the midline, halfway to two-thirds the distance from the infundibular recess to the mammillary bodies.

The floor can be perforated using one of several described techniques including use of the endoscope itself,[14,88] use of a semirigid stylet,[89] bipolar or monopolar coagulation,[90,91] suction cutting devices, and a spreading instrument.[47,92] There are advantages and disadvantages to each method. Perforation using the scope itself is thought to decrease the risk of vascular injury; however, the force required to penetrate the thickened floor can potentially cause hypothalamic injury. Use of a rigid instrument, such as closed biopsy forceps or Decq forceps,[93] which can be opened under direct vision, is less traumatic and allows direct vision during perforation; however, there is a risk of vascular injury if the forceps are opened after penetration (with avulsion of perforators) or if they are closed before withdrawal. Typically, the opening is enlarged by inflating a balloon of a 3F Fogarty catheter to achieve an adequate fenestration size of 3 to 6 mm. The interpeduncular and prepontine cisterns are inspected through the ventriculostomy and, if Liliequist's membrane is present, it is fenestrated. After withdrawing the endoscope, the brain tract is filled with Gelfoam (Upjohn, Kalamazoo, MI) to prevent egress and potential accumulation of subdural fluid.

The outcome after ETV is clearly related to patient selection.[12,23,31,51,59,63,67,73,94–106] In patients with obstruction at the level of the cerebral aqueduct, success rates are generally high and have been reported at up to 90%.[9,51,63] Outcomes are generally poorer in those with communicating types including postinfectious or post-hemorrhagic hydrocephalus. In a retrospective analysis of the operative success and long-term reliability of ETV in 203 patients with follow-up for up to 22.6 years,[12] the overall probability of success (failure defined as shunt insertion, ETV revision, or death) was 89%. Compared with the Canadian study, this study supported an association between the surgical success and the individual operating surgeon (odds ratios for success, 0.44–1.47 relative to the mean of 1.0, $P = .08$). As mentioned, the only statistically significant factor associated with long-term reliability was age, with the statistical model predicting the following reliability at 1 year after insertion: at 0 to 1 month of age, 31% (14%–53%); at 1 to 6 months of age, 50% (32%–68%); at 6 to 24 months of age, 71% (55%–85%); and at more than 24 months of age, 84% (79%–89%). In this study, there was no support for an association between reliability and the diagnostic group (n = 181, P = .168) or a previous shunt. In the Canadian Pediatric Neurosurgery Study Group study,[45] the overall 1- and 5- year success rates for ETV were 65% and 52%, respectively. These slightly lower outcomes results can be explained by use of a different measure of success and failure: in this study, success was strictly defined by no further CSF diversion procedures, whereas others have used placement of a shunt as the definition of failure. In a study of 131 patients undergoing ETV,[107] at 1 year follow-up, 82.5% of 86 primary ETV and 80% of 45 secondary ETV were shunt free.

In the case of ETV for treatment of obstructions distal to the fourth ventricle, results have been mixed, which may be due to a variety of factors causing distal obstruction. Fourth ventricular outlet obstruction is most commonly associated with prior intraventricular hemorrhage or infection. In a retrospective analysis of patients with fourth ventricular outlet obstruction, ETV was successfully performed in 20 of 22 patients with a follow-up period 1 to 8 years (Mean 4.2 years).[19] There was a high failure rate in those younger than 6 months.

ETV may also be a safe and effective means of treating hydrocephalus in the older (greater than age 2 years) spina bifida population and offers the hope of long-term shunt independence for selected patients.[14] In one study, ETV was performed on 69 patients with hydrocephalus and myelomeningocele. Most of the patients had been previously shunted, although in 14 patients ETV was the initial treatment. Patient selection was based on preoperative imaging studies suggesting noncommunicating hydrocephalus. There were no serious complications and the overall success rate was 72%, although selecting only patients who had been previously shunted or who were older than 6 months at the time of endoscopy increased success to 80%. ETV success in the myelomeningocele population has clinical importance, as approximately 90% of those with myelomeningocele develop hydrocephalus requiring diversion.[108]

The reasons for failure after ETV are still poorly understood and likely multifactorial. In some cases, there is presumably a communicating component to the hydrocephalus, with clearance issues that cannot be addressed by bypassing an interventricular obstruction. These patients require shunt placement. Ventriculostomy closure has been identified for failure in some cases, offering the possibility for a second ETV procedure over shunting. This question was addressed in a retrospective analysis of 482 ETVs in pediatric patients from 2 Italian centers.[109] In the 40 patients undergoing a second operation after initial ETV failure, the stoma was found to be closed in 28 patients without underlying adhesion, to be open but with significant prepontine arachnoid adhesion in 8 patients, to be open without adhesions in 2 patients, to have a pinhole orifice in 1 patient, and to be closed with underlying adhesions in 1 patient. A second procedure allowed reopening of the stoma or lysis of adhesions in 35 of 40 patients, and this was effective 75% of the time. Of importance, age younger than 2 years at the time of the first procedure and arachnoid adhesions in the subarachnoid cisterns observed during the second procedure were the main negative prognostic factors for the success of a second ETV. This finding may support the strategy to shunt children younger than 2, and reserve ETV in the case of shunt failure after the age of 2 years. In the article by Kadrian and colleagues[12] that retrospectively analyzed 203 patients, there was no support for an association between reliability and the diagnostic group (n = 181, P = .168) or a previous shunt. Sixteen patients had ETV repeated but only 9 were repeated after at least 6 months. Of these, 4 procedures failed within a few weeks, and 2 patients were available for long-term follow-up. In the future, stent placement may decrease the incidence of stoma closure.

In developing countries where a dependence on shunts is considered dangerous, ETV combined with choroid plexus coagulation (CPC) may be the best option for treating hydrocephalus in infants, particularly for those with non-postinfectious hydrocephalus and myelomeningocele. Warf[104,105,110,111] prospectively studied bilateral CPC in combination with ETV in 266 patients, and ETV alone in 284 patients. Of importance, 81% were younger than 1 year. The hydrocephalus was postinfectious in 320 patients, non-postinfectious in 152, and associated with myelomeningocele in 73. Overall, the success rate of ETV-CPC (66%) was superior to that of ETV alone (47%) among infants younger than 1 year (P<.0001). The ETV-CPC combined procedure was superior in patients with a myelomeningocele (76% compared with 35% success, P = .0045) and those with non-postinfectious hydrocephalus (70% compared with 38% success, P = .0025). For patients at least 1 year old, there was no difference between the 2 procedures (80% success for each, P = 1.0000).

Aqueductoplasty

In the treatment of aqueductal stenosis, anatomic variations can often render ETV a dangerous or impossible option. Cerebral aqueductoplasty has gained popularity as an effective treatment for membranous and short-segment stenosis of the cerebral aqueduct.[33,53,56,112–115] This procedure can be performed via a precoronal approach (burr hole placed 8 cm from nasion and 3 cm lateral to midline), passing through the lateral ventricle, foramen of Monro, and third ventricle into the aqueduct, or via a suboccipital foramen magnum trans-fourth ventricle approach. The floor of the third ventricle and proximal aqueduct can be inspected with a 0°, 30°, or 70° endoscope. If the stenosis is located distally in the aqueduct and this cannot be visualized using a rigid scope, a steerable fiberscope can be used to inspect the aqueduct. Aqueductoplasty can be performed with the aid of a 2F or 3F Fogarty balloon catheter, which is gently passed into the stenosis and dilated. The tip of the catheter should be bent to enable passage through the distal aqueduct and fourth ventricle because the aqueduct is not straight, but curved (see **Fig. 2**B), and a straight catheter may damage the tectum.[115]

A foramen magnum trans-fourth ventricular approach may offer advantages compared with the more traditional anterior approach. The fourth ventricular approach does not traverse brain tissue, does not depend on ventricular dilatation, and is a straight approach with no pressure on structures of the foramen of Monro.[114]

The decision to treat aqueductal stenosis by ETV rather than aqueductoplasty depends on the anatomy of the individual patient and the experience and comfort of the endoscopist.

To address the benefit of an intra-aqueductal stent to ensure continued patency of the aqueduct following this procedure, Cinalli and colleagues[116] conducted a retrospective evaluation of the effectiveness of endoscopic aqueductoplasty performed alone or accompanied by placement of a stent in the treatment of isolated fourth ventricle in 7 patients with supratentorial shunts and loculated hydrocephalus. These investigators found placement of a stent to be more effective than aqueductoplasty alone in preventing the repeated occlusion of the aqueduct. Aqueductal stenting is also a good procedure for treatment of isolated fourth ventricle.[18,19,56,113] Stenting is indicated when an increased risk of restenosis is expected. The stent should be at least 6 cm or longer to prevent migration. An alternative fixation option is suturing the stent to the dura at the entry point.

Lamina Terminalis Fenestration

If abnormal anatomy makes ETV and/or aqueductoplasty too risky, lamina terminalis fenestration can be an option for the treatment of any obstruction proximal to the fourth ventricular outlet. This procedure is performed in the setting of a translucent lamina terminalis to enable identification of the anterior cerebral arteries. The burr hole is usually placed in the same location as an ETV. If the foramen of Monro is large, the lamina terminalis can be visualized with a rigid 0° scope. If the foramen is narrow, a flexible scope must be used to avoid fornix damage. The lamina terminalis is perforated in the same manner as ETV and the perforation enlarged as well by inflating a Fogarty balloon catheter. Care is taken to preserve the chiasm and anterior cerebral arteries.[33,117]

Septum Pellucidotomy

Fenestration of the septum pellucidum is indicated for treatment of a blocked foramen of Monro, leading to dilatation of an ipsilateral lateral ventricle (**Fig. 4**).[33,117,118] This procedure is successful only if the contralateral foramen of Monro is patent and there is no further distal obstruction. It is also indicated in the event of bilateral obstruction of both foramina of Monro (see **Fig. 4**B and C), in conjunction either with communication of one lateral ventricle with the third ventricle (foraminoplasty), or with placement of single ventriculoperitoneal shunt; this avoids the need to place either 2 shunts, or a "Y" connection of 2 ventricular catheters.

The entry point is typically 5 to 6 cm paramedian, and 1 cm anterior to the coronal suture. Some surgeons prefer to enter on the side of the smaller lateral ventricle, to avoid injury to the contralateral head of caudate nucleus following fenestration. Others advocate entering on the side of the dilated ventricle,[33,117,118] allowing easier initial access to the ventricular system. When using a free-hand technique, entering on the side of the dilated ventricle is easier. However, if the contralateral ventricle is compressed or slit-like, there is a possibility of injury to the contralateral head of the caudate nucleus when creating an opening in the septum. This possibility is minimized if the smaller ventricle is entered initially, as the fenestration is made into a large fluid space. The disadvantage to placing a burr hole on the side of the smaller ventricle is that with a free-hand technique, it is possible that the contralateral ventricle will inadvertently be entered. This possibility can be avoided by using navigation. For

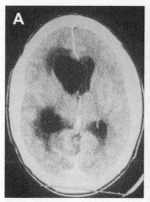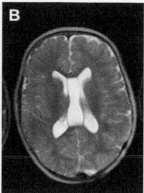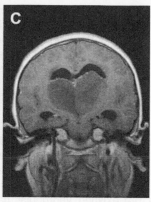

Fig. 4. Indications for septum pellucidotomy. Septum pellucidotomy is indicated in the setting of obstruction at the level of the foramen of Monro. Examples include unilateral foramen of Monro stenosis (*A*) treated with septum pellucidotomy alone, enlarged cavum septum pellucidum leading to bilateral foramen of Monro stenosis (*B*) treated with fenestration of both cavum membranes, and bithalamic tumor with obstruction of both foramina of Monro (*C*), which can be treated with septum pellucidotomy, and placement of unilateral shunt.

septum pellucidotomy, navigation is useful for determining the optimal entry point as well as the optimal point of septum fenestration.

The point of fenestration often depends on the individual anatomy. In some cases, there is a thin and avascular portion of the septum suitable for fenestration. Fenestration can be performed using monopolar coagulation with a hook instrument, or using blunt perforation.[118] The perforation can be enlarged with the aid of a Fogarty balloon catheter and scissors, or with monopolar, or bipolar diathermy. The fenestration size should be at least 1 cm in diameter; this is especially true in cases of thick septum, so as to avoid risk of ostomy closure.

Foraminoplasty

An alternative technique for treatment of isolated lateral ventricle is foraminoplasty.[119] This technique aims to restore the normal drainage pathway from the lateral ventricle into the third ventricle. The entry point is similar to that for ETV. The foramen of Monro is found by following the choroid plexus. The ependyma is coagulated and a spreading instrument inserted into the third ventricle anterior to the plexus, avoiding the fornix. Navigation improves safety. Dilatation with a Fogarty balloon is helpful.

Lysis of Intraventricular Adhesions

Neuroendoscopic management is an effective treatment for complex multi- and uni-loculated hydrocephalus, which has more traditionally been treated with multiple shunts, multiperforated catheters, stereotactic aspiration, or shunt placement and craniotomy with lysis of intraventricular

septations.[12,21,117,120,121] Multiple shunts are often unsuccessful due to increased risk of infection, obstruction, and hemorrhage associated with their removal.

Endoscopic treatment is extremely valuable in treating loculated ventricles and for communication of isolated CSF compartments. The goal is communication of all CSF spaces. Membrane lysis/fenestration is often combined with other traditional fenestration techniques including foramen of Monro reconstruction, septum pellucidotomy, septal wall removal, cyst wall fenestration, ETV, stenting between lateral and third ventricle, fourth ventriculostomy, and endoscopic shunt placement.

In an attempt to simplify cases of complex hydrocephalus using minimally invasive endoscopic techniques, Kadrian and Teo and colleagues[121] studied 114 patients treated endoscopically who presented with either more than one shunt and/or multiloculated hydrocephalus (47 patients), isolated lateral ventricle (25 patients), isolated fourth ventricle (20 patients), arachnoid cyst (15 patients), slit ventricle syndrome (4 patients) or cysticercosis (3 patients). The endoscopic procedures performed included cyst or membrane fenestration, septum pellucidotomy, ETV, aqueductal plasty with or without stent, endoscopic shunt placement, and retrieval and removal of cysticercotic cysts. Reduction to one shunt was possible in 72%, shunt independence in 28%, and only 11% required shunt revisions long-term.

There are numerous benefits to this approach. Multiloculated hydrocephalus is most commonly secondary to infection. Establishing CSF flow (a nidus for infection) and removal of shunts may be beneficial. With just one shunt, there are fewer opportunities for obstruction, malfunction, disconnection, and infection. Moreover, in patients with multiloculated hydrocephalus, it is easier to identify the source of shunt malfunction as compared with multiple shunts.

Practically speaking, the following principles should direct surgical approach: (1) the burr hole should be made in a position to make the cortical passage as short as possible, the endoscope will enter the largest cavity, and the trajectory will take the endoscope to the membrane that separates the 2 cavities that need to be joined; (2) if there is a pre-existing ventricular catheter that does not drain an isolated portion of the ventricle, then its tract can be used to enter the ventricle; (3) the trajectory should try to communicate as many cavities as possible; (4) as many fenestrations as possible should be made using a sharp technique.

Arachnoid Cysts

Optimal treatment of arachnoid cysts remains controversial. Options include no treatment, shunting, or fenestration via craniotomy with resection of cyst wall, stereotactic cyst fenestration, or endoscopic fenestration (**Fig. 5**). When cyst wall fenestration into the basal cisterns is contemplated, endoscopy is valuable due to its better visualization, magnification, angled perspective, and ability to maintain cyst distention during the procedure. Endoscopic management of arachnoid cysts has been extensively reported.[12,122–136] Greenfield and Souweidane[128] analyzed a prospectively generated database of 33 patients who underwent endoscopic fenestration of arachnoid cysts. Fenestration was successful as judged by cyst decompression and symptom resolution in 97%,

with only one initial failure that was successful after repeated endoscopic fenestration. Suprasellar cysts, which represent less than 10% of all intracranial arachnoid cysts, can be successfully treated endoscopically with good clinical outcome and low surgical morbidity. Ventriculo-cysto-cisternostomy should be attempted, but when the communication between the cyst and the cistern is considered too dangerous, ventriculo-cystostomy is acceptable.

Tumor-Related CSF Obstruction

Neuroendoscopy plays several roles in the surgical management of brain tumors and their occasional interference with CSF circulation.[33,102,117,137–146] Often, the CSF obstruction can be fully treated via endoscopic removal of the tumor causing the obstruction. Colloid cysts, benign lesions that arise from the velum interpositum or choroid plexus of the third ventricle, can produce hydrocephalus by obstruction of the foramina of Monro. Colloid cysts represent the ideal tumor for purely endoscopic excision (small with minimal vascularity).

Obstructive hydrocephalus is common with presentation of posterior fossa tumors. The incidence of hydrocephalus requiring CSF diversion following tumor resection remains at between 10% and 62%.[16,51,147–153] Due to the lack of prospective clinical trials, there is no consensus on proper perioperative management of this condition.[153] Pre-resectional hydrocephalus can be managed with an initial CSF diversional procedure such as ventricular drain or CSF shunt, or by resection alone. Postoperative shunt placement has historically been the management strategy for definitive treatment of communicating

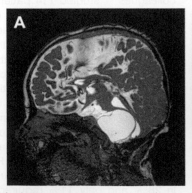
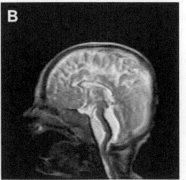

Fig. 5. Case example: large prepontine arachnoid cyst. A 26-week preterm female infant with grade 4 intraventricular hemorrhage developed post-hemorrhagic hydrocephalus and underwent shunt placement at age 4 weeks. She presented at age 7 months with pneumonia, respiratory distress, apnea, and poor feeding. MRI showed a large cyst anterior to the brainstem with severe thinning of her pons and medulla (A). She underwent endoscopic membrane fenestration through existing shunt tract, with improvement of symptoms within 24 hours. MRI scan 48 hours later (B) showed significant improvement of brainstem compression.

hydrocephalus. ETV has emerged as a compelling treatment strategy for CSF diversion both before and after resection. Tamburrini and colleagues[154] found that postoperative ETV placement in the setting of high ICP following removal of posterior fossa tumor was successful in 90% (27/30) of the patients. In a retrospective analysis of 59 children presenting with posterior fossa tumors and no (n = 16), mild,[49] moderate,[95] or severe[155] hydrocephalus, 37 (63%) underwent pre-resectional ETV with a high success rate for up to 7.5 years, with only 5 of 37 being failures.[156] Although no direct comparisons have been made, evidence appears to support ETV as a method for treatment of hydrocephalus associated with posterior fossa tumors, even after resection.

Intracranial Frameless Navigation

The combination of neuronavigation with neuroendoscopy improves safety and accuracy with such things as tumor biopsy, tumor resection, ETV, cyst wall fenestration, and ability to access small or slit ventricles. The usefulness of navigation in intracranial endoscopy has been extensively studied.[6,79,115,128,131,135,155,157–161] Navigation can be used to plan the correct entry point and trajectory, minimizing the potential for damage to the foramen of Monro and other brain tissue by reducing back-and-forth and side-to-side motion of the endoscope. The technique can be performed using a simple rigid endoscope through predetermined entry points and trajectories. Navigational tracking is most helpful in entering small ventricles, in approaching the posterior third ventricle when the foramen of Monro is narrow, and in selecting the best approach to colloid cysts. It is essential in some cystic lesions lacking clear landmarks, such as intraparenchymal cysts or multiloculated hydrocephalus.

COMPLICATIONS

Although neuroendoscopy has revolutionized the treatment of CSF disorders, specific complications occur due to risks inherent in the procedure and, sometimes, inexperience. Attempts should be made to avoid these problems. These complications have been extensively reviewed by experienced endoscopists, with suggestions made for their avoidance.[4,8,12,14,33,40,51,55,63,73,85,98,100,107,162–178]

Complications specific to ETV are best understood, and include bradycardia and asystole during manipulation of the third ventricular floor,[179] damage to the fornices with scope manipulation or poorly placed burr holes, hypothalamic pituitary axis damage,[173,176] damage to structures adjacent to the floor of the third ventricle including cranial nerves,[173] injury to major vessels resulting in subarachnoid hemorrhage[170] or ischemic stroke,[180] subdural hygroma or hematoma,[143,181] herniation,[51,181] remote intracranial hemorrhage,[42,169] infections,[42,173] and severe cognitive[182] and psychiatric sequelae.[163] Deaths associated with ETV have been reported acutely due to hemorrhage[4,42,45,54,68,165,173,183–186] and delayed from infection,[173] and even late, after sudden closure of the third ventriculostomy many months or years after a successful procedure. In a retrospective review of 131 patients undergoing ETV with a minimum follow-up duration of 1 year, serious complications after ETV occurred more frequently in patients who presented at the time of shunt malfunction (14 of 45 patients, 31%) compared with patients who underwent primary ETV (7 of 86 patients, 8%), (P = .02).[107] In a retrospective study of 203 patients for up to 22.6 years, infections were observed in 4.9%, transient major complications in 7.2%, and major and permanent complications in 1.1%.[12] Complications specifically related to aqueductoplasty include transient vertical diplopia or upgaze weakness.[114]

Complications in endoscopic surgery are not negligible even in experienced hands. Cinalli and colleagues[165] recently analyzed the complications recorded in a prospectively collected database of pediatric patients undergoing neuroendoscopic procedures. Complications occurred in 32 of 231 (13.8%) procedures performed for the management of obstructive hydrocephalus (137 patients), multiloculated hydrocephalus (53 patients), arachnoid cysts (29 patients), and intraventricular tumors (12 patients). Among complications, subdural hygroma occurred in 11 cases, CSF infection in 11, CSF leak in 9, intraventricular hemorrhages in 2, technical failures in 7, subcutaneous CSF collection in 1, thalamic contusion in 1, and transient akinetic mutism in 1 patient who died 6 months following the procedure. Three patients developed permanent disability as a consequence of surgical complication (1.3%).

Many of these complications can be avoided with experience and careful technique. As a general rule, the endoscope should not be used to find the ventricle. Even though the ventricle may be grossly dilated, inaccurate placement of an endoscope, unlike a fine brain needle, is not well tolerated. Side-to-side movements of the scope can tear bridging veins or stretch neural structures, and should be minimized. One should always check to see that there is an adequate outflow mechanism to allow for egress of the irrigation fluid. One should make sure that the edges of the rigid scope are blunt and rounded. Alternatively, when using a flexible scope one should check to ensure that the scope is in the neutral position before removal. One should use a peel-away sheath if the procedure requires multiple passages of the endoscope. Fornix damage can be avoided with optimal burr hole placement, and if the contralateral ventricle is entered, it should not be used for ETV. If the foramen of Monro is small, it should be enlarged before the procedure. Hypothalamic damage can be avoided by penetrating the third ventricular floor away from infundibular recess in the midline. Cranial neuropathies can be avoided by staying in the midline and recognizing and identifying the relevant anatomy before making any definitive maneuvers. Subdural hygromas can be avoided by expanding ventricle before removal of scope, plugging the cortical hole with Gelfoam, and avoiding ventricular drainage. CSF should be drained from cysts and ventricles slowly, and once the procedure has been accomplished, the cavities should be refilled to minimize the risk of subdural collections.

SUMMARY AND FUTURE DIRECTIONS

When faced with the patient with hydrocephalus, the ideal goal is to restore normal CSF hydrodynamics to a near physiologic state, with a safe procedure that is likely to not fail or require revision. To meet this goal, minimally invasive techniques, particularly neuroendoscopic procedures, have emerged as a therapy that is superior to shunting in appropriately selected patients. The potential applications for endoscopic techniques are rapidly growing, and this has had a dramatic effect on the treatment of nearly all disorders of CSF circulation. The main role of the endoscope in neurosurgery continues to reside in removing obstructions of CSF flow and/or diverting flow, with little disruption of normal brain tissue. Using these minimally invasive techniques, shunts can often be avoided or removed. For the patient this may mean less pain, shorter hospital stays, and improved outcome. Future investigations in this area should focus on better elaborating postoperative patient outcomes, providing a more thorough understanding about patient selection and factors that predict treatment failure, and undertaking formal, prospective evaluations of the comparative efficacy of endoscopic procedures compared with traditional shunting and open craniotomy operations.

REFERENCES

1. Nulsen F, Spitz E. Treatment of hydrocephalus by direct shunt from ventricle to jugular vein. Surg Forum 1952;399–403.

2. Hoffmann KT, Lehmann TN, Baumann C, et al. CSF flow imaging in the management of third ventriculostomy with a reversed fast imaging with steady-state precession sequence. Eur Radiol 2003;13:1432–7.

3. Foroutan M, Mafee MF, Dujovny M. Third ventriculostomy, phase-contrast cine MRI and endoscopic techniques. Neurol Res 1998;20:443–8.

4. Crandon IW, Ramcharan R, Harding H, et al. Neuroendoscopy in Jamaica. West Indian Med J 2005;54:34–7.

5. Sandberg DI. Endoscopic management of hydrocephalus in pediatric patients: a review of indications, techniques, and outcomes. J Child Neurol 2008;23:550–60.

6. Souweidane MM, Hoffman CE, Schwartz TH. Transcavum interforniceal endoscopic surgery of the third ventricle. J Neurosurg Pediatr 2008;2:231–6.

7. Stan H, Popa C, Iosif A, et al. Combined endoscopically guided third ventriculostomy with prepontine cistern placement of the ventricular catheter in a ventriculo-peritoneal shunt: technical note. Minim Invasive Neurosurg 2007;50:247–50.

8. van Beijnum J, Hanlo PW, Fischer K, et al. Laser-assisted endoscopic third ventriculostomy: long-term results in a series of 202 patients. Neurosurgery 2008;62:437–43 [discussion: 443–4].

9. Jones RF, Kwok BC, Stening WA, et al. The current status of endoscopic third ventriculostomy in the management of non-communicating hydrocephalus. Minim Invasive Neurosurg 1994;37:28–36.

10. Jones RF, Kwok BC, Stening WA, et al. Third ventriculostomy for hydrocephalus associated with spinal dysraphism: indications and contraindications. Eur J Pediatr Surg 1996;6(Suppl 1):5–6.

11. Jones RF, Stening WA, Brydon M. Endoscopic third ventriculostomy. Neurosurgery 1990;26:86–91 [discussion: 91–2].

12. Kadrian D, van Gelder J, Florida D, et al. Long-term reliability of endoscopic third ventriculostomy. Neurosurgery 56 2005 1271–8. [reprint in Neurosurgery 2008;62 (Suppl 2):614–21; PMID: 18596443] [discussion: 1278].

13. Levine NB, Tanaka T, Jones BV, et al. Minimally invasive management of a traumatic artery aneurysm resulting from shaken baby syndrome [see comment]. Pediatr Neurosurg 2004;40:128–31.

14. Teo C, Jones R. Management of hydrocephalus by endoscopic third ventriculostomy in patients with myelomeningocele. Pediatr Neurosurg 1996;25:57–63 [discussion: 63].

15. Decq P, Le Guerinel C, Sol JC, et al. Chiari I malformation: a rare cause of noncommunicating hydrocephalus treated by third ventriculostomy. J Neurosurg 2001;95:783–90.

16. Fritsch MJ, Doerner L, Kienke S, et al. Hydrocephalus in children with posterior fossa tumors: role of

endoscopic third ventriculostomy. J Neurosurg 2005;103:40–2.

17. Longatti P, Fiorindi A, Feletti A, et al. Endoscopic opening of the foramen of Magendie using transaqueductal navigation for membrane obstruction of the fourth ventricle outlets. Technical note. J Neurosurg 2006;105:924–7.

18. Mohanty A. Endoscopic options in the management of isolated fourth ventricles. Case report. J Neurosurg 2005;103:73–8.

19. Mohanty A, Biswas A, Satish S, et al. Efficacy of endoscopic third ventriculostomy in fourth ventricular outlet obstruction. Neurosurgery 2008;63:905–13 [discussion: 913–4].

20. Oertel JMK, Mondorf Y, Gaab MR. Endoscopic third ventriculostomy in obstructive hydrocephalus due to giant basilar artery aneurysm. J Neurosurg 2009;110:14–8.

21. Teo CM, Burson TM, Misra SM. Endoscopic treatment of the trapped fourth ventricle. Neurosurgery 1999;44:1257–61.

22. Amini A, Schmidt RH. Endoscopic third ventriculostomy in a series of 36 adult patients. Neurosurg Focus 2005;19:E9.

23. Feng H, Huang G, Liao X, et al. Endoscopic third ventriculostomy in the management of obstructive hydrocephalus: an outcome analysis. J Neurosurg 2004;100:626–33.

24. Figaji AA, Fieggen AG, Peter JC. Endoscopic third ventriculostomy in tuberculous meningitis [see comment]. Childs Nerv Syst 2003;19:217–25.

25. Figaji AA, Fieggen AG, Peter JC. Air encephalography for hydrocephalus in the era of neuroendoscopy. Childs Nerv Syst 2005;21:559–65.

26. Gangemi M, Maiuri F, Buonamassa S, et al. Endoscopic third ventriculostomy in idiopathic normal pressure hydrocephalus. Neurosurgery 2004;55:129–34 [discussion: 134].

27. Gangemi M, Maiuri F, Naddeo M, et al. Endoscopic third ventriculostomy in idiopathic normal pressure hydrocephalus: an Italian multicenter study. Neurosurgery 2008;63:62–7 [discussion: 67–9].

28. Garg A, Suri A, Chandra PS, et al. Endoscopic third ventriculostomy: 5 years' experience at the All India Institute of Medical Sciences. Pediatr Neurosurg 2009;45:1–5.

29. Hailong F, Guangfu H, Haibin T, et al. Endoscopic third ventriculostomy in the management of communicating hydrocephalus: a preliminary study. J Neurosurg 2008;109:923–30.

30. Hellwig D, Grotenhuis JA, Tirakotai W, et al. Endoscopic third ventriculostomy for obstructive hydrocephalus. Neurosurg Rev 2005;28:1–34 [discussion: 35–8].

31. Iantosca MR, Hader WJ, Drake JM. Results of endoscopic third ventriculostomy. Neurosurg Clin N Am 2004;15:67–75.

32. Kwiek SJ, Mandera M, Baowski P, et al. Endoscopic third ventriculostomy for hydrocephalus: early and late efficacy in relation to aetiology. Acta Neurochir (Wien) 2003;145:181–4.

33. Oertel JMK, Baldauf J, Schroeder HWS, et al. Endoscopic options in children: experience with 134 procedures. J Neurosurg Pediatr 2009;3:81–9.

34. Paladino J, Rotim K, Stimac D, et al. Endoscopic third ventriculostomy with ultrasonic contact microprobe. Minim Invasive Neurosurg 2000;43:132–4.

35. Ray P, Jallo GI, Kim RYH, et al. Endoscopic third ventriculostomy for tumor-related hydrocephalus in a pediatric population. Neurosurg Focus 2005;19:E8.

36. Rekate HL. Selecting patients for endoscopic third ventriculostomy. Neurosurg Clin N Am 2004;15:39–49.

37. Siomin V, Cinalli G, Grotenhuis A, et al. Endoscopic third ventriculostomy in patients with cerebrospinal fluid infection and/or hemorrhage. J Neurosurg 2002;97:519–24.

38. Siomin V, Weiner H, Wisoff J, et al. Repeat endoscopic third ventriculostomy: is it worth trying? Childs Nerv Syst 2001;17:551–5.

39. Koch D, Wagner W. Endoscopic third ventriculostomy in infants of less than 1 year of age: which factors influence the outcome? Childs Nerv Syst 2004;20:405–11.

40. Kulkarni AV, Drake JM, Mallucci CL, et al. Canadian Pediatric Neurosurgery Study G: Endoscopic third ventriculostomy in the treatment of childhood hydrocephalus. J Pediatr 2009;155:254–9, e251.

41. Wagner W, Koch D. Mechanisms of failure after endoscopic third ventriculostomy in young infants. J Neurosurg 2005;103:43–9.

42. Buxton N, Cartmill M, Vloeberghs M. Endoscopic third ventriculostomy: outcome analysis of 100 consecutive procedures [see comment]. Neurosurgery 1999;45:957–9.

43. Di Rocco C, Cinalli G, Massimi L, et al. Endoscopic third ventriculostomy in the treatment of hydrocephalus in pediatric patients. Adv Tech Stand Neurosurg 2006;31:119–219.

44. Fritsch MJ, Kienke S, Ankermann T, et al. Endoscopic third ventriculostomy in infants. J Neurosurg 2005;103:50–3.

45. Drake JM, Canadian Pediatric Neurosurgery Study G. Endoscopic third ventriculostomy in pediatric patients: the Canadian experience. Neurosurgery 2007;60:881–6 [discussion: 881–6].

46. Lipina R, Reguli S, Dolezilova V, et al. Endoscopic third ventriculostomy for obstructive hydrocephalus in children younger than 6 months of age: is it a first-choice method? Childs Nerv Syst 2008;24:1021–7.

47. Baldauf J, Oertel J, Gaab MR, et al. Endoscopic third ventriculostomy in children younger than 2 years of age. Childs Nerv Syst 2007;23:623–6.

48. Bech-Azeddine R, Nielsen OA, Logager VB, et al. Lumbar elastance and resistance to CSF outflow correlated to patency of the cranial subarachnoid space and clinical outcome of endoscopic third ventriculostomy in obstructive hydrocephalus. Minim Invasive Neurosurg 2007;50:189–94.

49. Beems T, Grotenhuis JA. Is the success rate of endoscopic third ventriculostomy age-dependent? An analysis of the results of endoscopic third ventriculostomy in young children. Childs Nerv Syst 2002;18:605–8.

50. Boschert J, Hellwig D, Krauss JK. Endoscopic third ventriculostomy for shunt dysfunction in occlusive hydrocephalus: long-term follow up and review [see comment]. J Neurosurg 2003;98:1032–9.

51. Brockmeyer D, Abtin K, Carey L, et al. Endoscopic third ventriculostomy: an outcome analysis. Pediatr Neurosurg 1998;28:236–40.

52. Civelek E, Cansever T, Karasu A, et al. Chronic subdural hematoma after endoscopic third ventriculostomy: case report. Turk Neurosurg 2007;17:289–93.

53. da Silva LRF, Cavalheiro S, Zymberg ST. Endoscopic aqueductoplasty in the treatment of aqueductal stenosis. Childs Nerv Syst 2007;23:1263–8.

54. Drake J, Chumas P, Kestle J, et al. Late rapid deterioration after endoscopic third ventriculostomy: additional cases and review of the literature. J Neurosurg 2006;105:118–26.

55. Dusick JR, McArthur DL, Bergsneider M. Success and complication rates of endoscopic third ventriculostomy for adult hydrocephalus: a series of 108 patients. Surg Neurol 2008;69:5–15.

56. Ersahin Y. Endoscopic aqueductoplasty. Childs Nerv Syst 2007;23:143–50.

57. Fukuhara T, Luciano MG. Clinical features of late-onset idiopathic aqueductal stenosis. Surg Neurol 2001;55:132–6 [discussion: 136–7].

58. Fukuhara T, Vorster SJ, Luciano MG. Risk factors for failure of endoscopic third ventriculostomy for obstructive hydrocephalus. Neurosurgery 2000;46:1100–9 [discussion: 1109–11].

59. Gangemi M, Mascari C, Maiuri F, et al. Long-term outcome of endoscopic third ventriculostomy in obstructive hydrocephalus. Minim Invasive Neurosurg 2007;50:265–9.

60. Garg AK, Suri A, Sharma BS, et al. Changes in cerebral perfusion hormone profile and cerebrospinal fluid flow across the third ventriculostomy after endoscopic third ventriculostomy in patients with aqueductal stenosis: a prospective study. Clinical article. J Neurosurg Pediatr 2009;3:29–36.

61. Gorayeb RP, Cavalheiro S, Zymberg ST. Endoscopic third ventriculostomy in children younger than 1 year of age. J Neurosurg 2004;100:427–9.

62. Grunert P, Charalampaki P, Hopf N, et al. The role of third ventriculostomy in the management of obstructive hydrocephalus. Minim Invasive Neurosurg 2003;46:16–21.

63. Hopf NJ, Grunert P, Fries G, et al. Endoscopic third ventriculostomy: outcome analysis of 100 consecutive procedures [see comment]. Neurosurgery 1999;44:795–804 [discussion: 804–6].

64. Husain M, Rastogi M, Jha DK. Endoscopic third ventriculostomy through the interfornicial space. Pediatr Neurosurg 2005;41:165–7.

65. Idowu O, Doherty A, Tiamiyu O. Initial experience with endoscopic third ventriculostomy in Nigeria, West Africa. Childs Nerv Syst 2008;24:253–5 [discussion: 257].

66. Javadpour M, Mallucci C, Brodbelt A, et al. The impact of endoscopic third ventriculostomy on the management of newly diagnosed hydrocephalus in infants. Pediatr Neurosurg 2001;35:131–5.

67. Koch-Wiewrodt D, Wagner W. Success and failure of endoscopic third ventriculostomy in young infants: are there different age distributions? Childs Nerv Syst 2006;22:1537–41.

68. Lipina R, Palecek T, Reguli S, et al. Death in consequence of late failure of endoscopic third ventriculostomy. Childs Nerv Syst 2007;23:815–9.

69. Mohanty A, Biswas A, Satish S, et al. Treatment options for Dandy-Walker malformation. J Neurosurg 2006;105:348–56.

70. Munch TN, Bech-Azeddine R, Boegeskov L, et al. Evaluation of the lumbar and ventricular infusion test in the diagnostic strategy of pediatric hydrocephalus and the therapeutic implications. Childs Nerv Syst 2007;23:67–71.

71. Rapana A, Bellotti A, Iaccarino C, et al. Intracranial pressure patterns after endoscopic third ventriculostomy. Preliminary experience. Acta Neurochir (Wien) 2004;146:1309–15 [discussion: 1315].

72. Rekate HL. Longstanding overt ventriculomegaly in adults: pitfalls in treatment with endoscopic third ventriculostomy. Neurosurg Focus 2007;22:E6.

73. Santamarta D, Diaz Alvarez A, Goncalves JM, et al. Outcome of endoscopic third ventriculostomy. Results from an unselected series with noncommunicating hydrocephalus. Acta Neurochir (Wien) 2005;147:377–82 [discussion: 382].

74. Tisell M. How should primary aqueductal stenosis in adults be treated? A review. Acta Neurol Scand 2005;111:145–53.

75. Tisell M, Almstrom O, Stephensen H, et al. How effective is endoscopic third ventriculostomy in treating adult hydrocephalus caused by primary aqueductal stenosis? Neurosurgery 2000;46:104–10 [discussion: 110–1].

76. Tisell M, Edsbagge M, Stephensen H, et al. Elastance correlates with outcome after endoscopic third ventriculostomy in adults with hydrocephalus caused by primary aqueductal stenosis. Neurosurgery 2002;50:70–7.

77. Yadav YR, Jaiswal S, Adam N, et al. Endoscopic third ventriculostomy in infants. Neurol India 2006; 54:161–3.

78. Kehler U, Regelsberger J, Gliemroth J, et al. Outcome prediction of third ventriculostomy: a proposed hydrocephalus grading system. Minim Invasive Neurosurg 2006;49:238–43.

79. Rohde V, Krombach GA, Struffert T, et al. Virtual MRI endoscopy: detection of anomalies of the ventricular anatomy and its possible role as a pre-surgical planning tool for endoscopic third ventriculostomy. Acta Neurochir (Wien) 2001;143: 1085–91.

80. St George E, Natarajan K, Sgouros S. Changes in ventricular volume in hydrocephalic children following successful endoscopic third ventriculostomy. Childs Nerv Syst 2004;20:834–8.

81. Longatti PL, Fiorindi A, Martinuzzi A. Failure of endoscopic third ventriculostomy in the treatment of idiopathic normal pressure hydrocephalus. Minim Invasive Neurosurg 2004;47:342–5.

82. Jenkinson MD, Hayhurst C, Al-Jumaily M, et al. The role of endoscopic third ventriculostomy in adult patients with hydrocephalus. J Neurosurg 2009; 110:861–6.

83. Costa Val JA. Minicraniotomy for endoscopic third ventriculostomy in babies: technical note with a 7-year-segment analysis. Childs Nerv Syst 2009;25: 357–9.

84. Devaux BC, Joly L-M, Page P, et al. Laser-assisted endoscopic third ventriculostomy for obstructive hydrocephalus: technique and results in a series of 40 consecutive cases. Laser Surg Med 2004; 34:368–78.

85. Ersahin Y, Arslan D. Complications of endoscopic third ventriculostomy. Childs Nerv Syst 2008;24: 943–8.

86. Sgaramella E, Castelli G, Sotgiu S. Chronic subdural collection after endoscopic third ventriculostomy. Acta Neurochir (Wien) 2004;146:529–30.

87. Kanner A, Hopf NJ, Grunert P. The "optimal" burr hole position for endoscopic third ventriculostomy: results from 31 stereotactically guided procedures. Minim Invasive Neurosurg 2000;43:187–9.

88. El-Dawlatly AA, Murshid W, El-Khwsky F. Endoscopic third ventriculostomy: a study of intracranial pressure vs. haemodynamic changes. Minim Invasive Neurosurg 1999;42:198–200.

89. Wellons JC 3rd, Bagley CA, George TM. A simple and safe technique for endoscopic third ventriculocisternostomy. Pediatr Neurosurg 1999;30: 219–23.

90. Chumas P, Sainte-Rose C, Cinalli G, et al. The management of hydrocephalus by endoscopic third ventriculostomy in pediatric patients with posterior fossa tumours—a preliminary study paper #725. Neurosurgery 1996;39:642–3.

91. Hellwig D, Haag R, Bartel V, et al. Application of new electrosurgical devices and probes in endoscopic neurosurgery. Neurol Res 1999;21:67–72.

92. Decq P, Le Guerinel C, Palfi S, et al. A new device for endoscopic third ventriculostomy [see comment]. J Neurosurg 2000;93:509–12.

93. Schroeder HWS, Nehlsen M. Value of high-definition imaging in neuroendoscopy. Neurosurg Rev 2009;32:303–8 [discussion: 308].

94. Balthasar AJ, Kort H, Cornips EM, et al. Analysis of the success and failure of endoscopic third ventriculostomy in infants less than 1 year of age. Childs Nerv Syst 2007;23:151–5.

95. Chugh A, Husain M, Gupta RK, et al. Surgical outcome of tuberculous meningitis hydrocephalus treated by endoscopic third ventriculostomy: prognostic factors and postoperative neuroimaging for functional assessment of ventriculostomy. J Neurosurg Pediatr 2009;3:371–7.

96. Drake JM, Kulkarni AV, Kestle J. Endoscopic third ventriculostomy versus ventriculoperitoneal shunt in pediatric patients: a decision analysis. Childs Nerv Syst 2009;25:467–72.

97. Greenfield JP, Hoffman C, Kuo E, et al. Intraoperative assessment of endoscopic third ventriculostomy success [see comment]. J Neurosurg Pediatr 2008;2:298–303.

98. Husain M, Jha D, Vatsal DK, et al. Neuro-endoscopic surgery—experience and outcome analysis of 102 consecutive procedures in a busy neurosurgical centre of India. Acta Neurochir (Wien) 2003; 145:369–75 [discussion: 375–6].

99. Jha DK, Mishra V, Choudhary A, et al. Factors affecting the outcome of neuroendoscopy in patients with tuberculous meningitis hydrocephalus: a preliminary study. Surg Neurol 2007;68: 35–41 [discussion: 41–2].

100. O'Brien DF, Javadpour M, Collins DR, et al. Endoscopic third ventriculostomy: an outcome analysis of primary cases and procedures performed after ventriculoperitoneal shunt malfunction. J Neurosurg 2005;103:393–400.

101. O'Brien DF, Seghedoni A, Collins DR, et al. Is there an indication for ETV in young infants in aetiologies other than isolated aqueduct stenosis? Childs Nerv Syst 2006;22:1565–72.

102. Souweidane MM. Endoscopic management of pediatric brain tumors. Neurosurg Focus 2005;18:E1.

103. Takahashi Y. Long-term outcome and neurologic development after endoscopic third ventriculostomy versus shunting during infancy. Childs Nerv Syst 2006;22:1591–602.

104. Warf BC. Comparison of endoscopic third ventriculostomy alone and combined with choroid plexus cauterization in infants younger than 1 year of age: a prospective study in 550 African children. J Neurosurg 2005;103:475–81.

105. Warf BC, Campbell JW. Combined endoscopic third ventriculostomy and choroid plexus cauterization as primary treatment of hydrocephalus for infants with myelomeningocele: long-term results of a prospective intent-to-treat study in 115 East African infants. J Neurosurg Pediatr 2008;2: 310–6.

106. Wiewrodt D, Schumacher R, Wagner W. Hygromas after endoscopic third ventriculostomy in the first year of life: incidence, management and outcome in a series of 34 patients. Childs Nerv Syst 2008; 24:57–63.

107. Hader WJ, Walker RL, Myles ST, et al. Complications of endoscopic third ventriculostomy in previously shunted patients. Neurosurgery 2008;63: ONS168–74 [discussion: ONS174–5].

108. Dias MS, McLone DG. Hydrocephalus in the child with dysraphism. Neurosurg Clin N Am 1993;4: 715–26.

109. Peretta P, Cinalli G, Spennato P, et al. Long-term results of a second endoscopic third ventriculostomy in children: retrospective analysis of 40 cases. Neurosurgery 2009;65:539–47.

110. Warf BC. Hydrocephalus in Uganda: the predominance of infectious origin and primary management with endoscopic third ventriculostomy. J Neurosurg 2005;102:1–15.

111. Warf BC. Endoscopic third ventriculostomy and choroid plexus cauterization for pediatric hydrocephalus. Clin Neurosurg 2007;54:78–82.

112. Gawish I, Reisch R, Perneczky A. Endoscopic aqueductoplasty through a tailored craniocervical approach [see comment]. J Neurosurg 2005;103: 778–82.

113. Hayashi N, Hamada H, Hirashima Y, et al. Clinical features in patients requiring reoperation after failed endoscopic procedures for hydrocephalus. Minim Invasive Neurosurg 2000;43:181–6.

114. Sansone JM, Iskandar BJ. Endoscopic cerebral aqueductoplasty: a trans-fourth ventricle approach [see comment]. J Neurosurg 2005;103:388–92.

115. Schroeder HW, Gaab MR. Endoscopic aqueductoplasty: technique and results. Neurosurgery 1999; 45:508–15 [discussion: 515–8].

116. Cinalli G, Spennato P, Savarese L, et al. Endoscopic aqueductoplasty and placement of a stent in the cerebral aqueduct in the management of isolated fourth ventricle in children [see comment]. J Neurosurg 2006;104:21–7.

117. Cappabianca P, Cinalli G, Gangemi M, et al. Application of neuroendoscopy to intraventricular lesions. Neurosurgery 2008;62(Suppl 2):575–97 [discussion: 597–8].

118. Oertel JMK, Schroeder HWS, Gaab MR. Endoscopic stomy of the septum pellucidum: indications, technique, and results. Neurosurgery 2009; 64:482–91 [discussion: 491–3].

119. Mori H, Koike T, Fujimoto T, et al. Endoscopic stent placement for treatment of secondary bilateral occlusion of the Monro foramina following endoscopic third ventriculostomy in a patient with aqueductal stenosis. Case report. J Neurosurg 2007; 107:416–20.

120. Johnston I, Teo C. Disorders of CSF hydrodynamics. Childs Nerv Syst 2000;16:776–99.

121. Kadrian DS, Teo C. Endoscopic management of complex hydrocephalus. ANZ J Surg 2002;72 (Suppl):A61.

122. Buxton N, Vloeberghs M, Punt J. Flexible neuroendoscopic treatment of suprasellar arachnoid cysts. Br J Neurosurg 1999;13:316–8.

123. Chernov MF, Kamikawa S, Yamane F, et al. Double-endoscopic approach for management of convexity arachnoid cyst: case report. Surg Neurol 2004;61:483–6 [discussion: 486–7].

124. Cincu R, Agrawal A, Eiras J. Intracranial arachnoid cysts: current concepts and treatment alternatives. Clin Neurol Neurosurg 2007;109:837–43.

125. Di Rocco F, Yoshino M, Oi S. Neuroendoscopic transventricular ventriculocystostomy in treatment for intracranial cysts. J Neurosurg 2005;103: 54–60.

126. Ersahin Y, Kesikci H. Endoscopic management of quadrigeminal arachnoid cysts. Childs Nerv Syst 2009;25:569–76.

127. Gangemi M, Colella G, Magro F, et al. Suprasellar arachnoid cysts: endoscopy versus microsurgical cyst excision and shunting. Br J Neurosurg 2007; 21:276–80.

128. Greenfield JP, Souweidane MM. Endoscopic management of intracranial cysts. Neurosurg Focus 2005;19:E7.

129. Inamasu J, Ohira T, Nakamura Y, et al. Endoscopic ventriculo-cystostomy for non-communicating hydrocephalus secondary to quadrigeminal cistern arachnoid cyst. Acta Neurol Scand 2003;107: 67–71.

130. Isik U, Ozek MM. Endoscopic treatment of in utero diagnosed suprasellar arachnoid cyst and development of salt wasting. Minim Invasive Neurosurg 2007;50:243–6.

131. Karabatsou K, Hayhurst C, Buxton N, et al. Endoscopic management of arachnoid cysts: an advancing technique. J Neurosurg 2007;106: 455–62.

132. Pradilla G, Jallo G. Arachnoid cysts: case series and review of the literature. Neurosurg Focus 2007;22:E7.

133. Rangel-Castilla L, Torres-Corzo J, Vecchia RRD, et al. Coexistent intraventricular abnormalities in periventricular giant arachnoid cysts. J Neurosurg Pediatr 2009;3:225–31.

134. Sood S, Schuhmann MU, Cakan N, et al. Endoscopic fenestration and coagulation shrinkage of

suprasellar arachnoid cysts. Technical note. J Neurosurg 2005;102:127–33.

135. Van Beijnum J, Hanlo PW, Han KS, et al. Navigated laser-assisted endoscopic fenestration of a suprasellar arachnoid cyst in a 2-year-old child with bobble-head doll syndrome [Case report]. J Neurosurg 2006;104:348–51.

136. Wang JC, Heier L, Souweidane MM, et al. Advances in the endoscopic management of suprasellar arachnoid cysts in children. J Neurosurg 2004;100:418–26 [erratum appears in J Neurosurg 2004;101(Suppl 1):123].

137. Greenlee JD, Teo C, Ghahreman A, et al. Purely endoscopic resection of colloid cysts. Neurosurgery Supplement 2008;62(3):51–6.

138. Mobbs R, Teo C. Endoscopic assisted posterior fossa decompression. J Clin Neurosci 2001;8: 343–4.

139. Mobbs RJ, Nakaji P, Szkandera BJ, et al. Endoscopic assisted posterior decompression for spinal neoplasms. J Clin Neurosci 2002;9:437–9.

140. Ong BC, Gore PA, Donnellan MB, et al. Endoscopic sublabial transmaxillary approach to the rostral middle fossa. Neurosurgery Supplement 2008;62(3):30–7.

141. Teo C. Endoscopy allows a keyhole approach to many skull base tumors. Neurosurgery 1998;43: 713.

142. Teo C, Greenlee JDW. Application of endoscopy to third ventricular tumors. Clin Neurosurg 2005;52: 24–8.

143. Teo C, Nakaji P. Neuro-oncologic applications of endoscopy. Neurosurg Clin N Am 2004;15: 89–103.

144. Teo C. Endoscopic-assisted tumor and neurovascular procedures. Clin Neurosurg 2000;46:515–25.

145. Teo C. Application of endoscopy to the surgical management of craniopharyngiomas. Childs Nerv Syst 2005;21:696–700.

146. Teo CMD, Siu TMD, Nakaji PMD. Surgical management of brainstem gliomas. Contemp Neurosurg 2005;27:1–7.

147. Due-Tonnessen BJ, Helseth E. Management of hydrocephalus in children with posterior fossa tumors: role of tumor surgery. Pediatr Neurosurg 2007;43:92–6.

148. Morelli D, Pirotte B, Lubansu A, et al. Persistent hydrocephalus after early surgical management of posterior fossa tumors in children: is routine preoperative endoscopic third ventriculostomy justified? J Neurosurg 2005;103:247–52.

149. Riva-Cambrin J, Detsky AS, Lamberti-Pasculli M, et al. Predicting postresection hydrocephalus in pediatric patients with posterior fossa tumors. J Neurosurg Pediatr 2009;3:378–85.

150. Ruggiero C, Cinalli G, Spennato P, et al. Endoscopic third ventriculostomy in the treatment of hydrocephalus in posterior fossa tumors in children. Childs Nerv Syst 2004;20:828–33.

151. Sainte-Rose C, Cinalli G, Roux FE, et al. Management of hydrocephalus in pediatric patients with posterior fossa tumors: the role of endoscopic third ventriculostomy. J Neurosurg 2001;95:791–7.

152. Santos de Oliveira R, Barros Juca CE, Valera ET, et al. Hydrocephalus in posterior fossa tumors in children. Are there factors that determine a need for permanent cerebrospinal fluid diversion? Childs Nerv Syst 2008;24:1397–403.

153. Schijman E, Peter JC, Rekate HL, et al. Management of hydrocephalus in posterior fossa tumors: how, what, when? Childs Nerv Syst 2004;20:192–4.

154. Tamburrini G, Pettorini BL, Massimi L, et al. Endoscopic third ventriculostomy: the best option in the treatment of persistent hydrocephalus after posterior cranial fossa tumour removal? Childs Nerv Syst 2008;24:1405–12.

155. Buxton N, Cartmill M, Buxton N, et al. Neuroendoscopy combined with frameless neuronavigation [comment]. Br J Neurosurg 2000;14:600–1.

156. Bhatia R, Tahir M, Chandler CL. The management of hydrocephalus in children with posterior fossa tumours: the role of pre-resectional endoscopic third ventriculostomy. Pediatr Neurosurg 2009;45: 186–91.

157. Broggi G, Dones I, Ferroli P, et al. Image guided neuroendoscopy for third ventriculostomy. Acta Neurochir (Wien) 2000;142:893–8 [discussion: 898–9].

158. Krombach A, Rohde V, Haage P, et al. Virtual endoscopy combined with intraoperative neuronavigation for planning of endoscopic surgery in patients with occlusive hydrocephalus and intracranial cysts. Neuroradiology 2002;44:279–85.

159. Riegel T, Alberti O, Hellwig D, et al. Operative management of third ventriculostomy in cases of thickened, non-translucent third ventricular floor: technical note. Minim Invasive Neurosurg 2001; 44:65–9.

160. Rohde V, Reinges MH, Krombach GA, et al. The combined use of image-guided frameless stereotaxy and neuroendoscopy for the surgical management of occlusive hydrocephalus and intracranial cysts. Br J Neurosurg 1998;12:531–8.

161. Wagner W, Gaab MR, Schroeder HW, et al. Experiences with cranial neuronavigation in pediatric neurosurgery. Pediatr Neurosurg 1999;31:231–6.

162. Beems T, Grotenhuis JA. Long-term complications and definition of failure of neuroendoscopic procedures. Childs Nerv Syst 2004;20:868–77.

163. Benabarre A, Ibanez J, Boget T, et al. Neuropsychological and psychiatric complications in endoscopic third ventriculostomy: a clinical case report [see comment]. J Neurol Neurosurg Psychiatr 2001;71:268–71.

164. Bullivant KJ, Hader W, Hamilton M. A pediatric experience with endoscopic third ventriculostomy for hydrocephalus. Can J Neurosci Nurs 2009;31: 16–9.

165. Cinalli G, Spennato P, Ruggiero C, et al. Complications following endoscopic intracranial procedures in children. Childs Nerv Syst 2007;23:633–44.

166. Di Rocco C, Massimi L, Tamburrini G. Shunts vs endoscopic third ventriculostomy in infants: are there different types and/or rates of complications? A review. Childs Nerv Syst 2006;22:1573–89.

167. Ganjoo P, Sethi S, Tandon MS, et al. Incidence and pattern of intraoperative hemodynamic response to endoscopic third ventriculostomy. Neurol India 2009;57:162–5.

168. Jamjoom AB, Jamjoom ZA, Ur Rahman N. Low rate of shunt revision in tumoural obstructive hydrocephalus. Acta Neurochir (Wien) 1998;140:595–7.

169. Kim B-S, Jallo GI, Kothbauer K, et al. Chronic subdural hematoma as a complication of endoscopic third ventriculostomy. Surg Neurol 2004; 62:64–8 [discussion: 68].

170. McLaughlin MR, Wahlig JB, Kaufmann AM, et al. Traumatic basilar aneurysm after endoscopic third ventriculostomy: case report [see comment]. Neurosurgery 1997;41:1400–3 [discussion: 1403–4].

171. Navarro R, Gil-Parra R, Reitman AJ, et al. Endoscopic third ventriculostomy in children: early and late complications and their avoidance. Childs Nerv Syst 2006;22:506–13.

172. O'Brien DF, Hayhurst C, Pizer B, et al. Outcomes in patients undergoing single-trajectory endoscopic third ventriculostomy and endoscopic biopsy for midline tumors presenting with obstructive hydrocephalus. J Neurosurg 2006;105:219–26.

173. Schroeder HWS, Niendorf W-R, Gaab MR. Complications of endoscopic third ventriculostomy. J Neurosurg 2002;96:1032–40.

174. Sgaramella E, Sotgiu S, Crotti FM. Overdrainage after endoscopic third ventriculostomy: an unusual case of chronic subdural hematoma—case report and review of the literature. Minim Invasive Neurosurg 2003;46:354–6.

175. Sleep TE, Elsas F. Strabismus after endoscopic third ventriculostomy. J AAPOS 2007;11:195–6.

176. Teo C, Rahman S, Boop FA, et al. Complications of endoscopic neurosurgery. Childs Nerv Syst 1996; 12:248–53 [discussion: 253].

177. Warf BC. Comparison of 1-year outcomes for the Chhabra and Codman-Hakim Micro Precision shunt systems in Uganda: a prospective study in 195 children [see comment]. J Neurosurg 2005;102:358–62.

178. Woodworth G, McGirt MJ, Thomas G, et al. Prior CSF shunting increases the risk of endoscopic third ventriculostomy failure in the treatment of obstructive hydrocephalus in adults. Neurol Res 2007;29:27–31.

179. Handler MH, Abbott R, Lee M. A near-fatal complication of endoscopic third ventriculostomy: case report. Neurosurgery 1994;35:525–7 [discussion: 527–8].

180. Buxton N, Punt J. Cerebral infarction after neuroendoscopic third ventriculostomy: case report. [see comment]. Neurosurgery 2000;46:999–1001 [discussion: 1001–2].

181. Baldauf J, Oertel J, Gaab MR, et al. Endoscopic third ventriculostomy for occlusive hydrocephalus caused by cerebellar infarction. Neurosurgery 2006;59:539–44 [discussion: 539–4].

182. Bonanni R, Carlesimo GA, Caltagirone C. Amnesia following endoscopic third ventriculostomy: a single case study. Eur Neurol 2004;51:118–20.

183. Constantini S, Siomin V. Re: Death after late failure of endoscopic third ventriculostomy: a potential solution [comment]. Neurosurgery 2005;56:E629.

184. Javadpour M, May P, Mallucci C. Sudden death secondary to delayed closure of endoscopic third ventriculostomy. Br J Neurosurg 2003;17:266–9.

185. Mobbs RJ, Vonau M, Davies MA. Death after late failure of endoscopic third ventriculostomy: a potential solution. [see comment]. Neurosurgery 2003;53:384–5 [discussion: 385–6].

186. Shono T, Natori Y, Morioka T, et al. Results of a long-term follow-up after neuroendoscopic biopsy procedure and third ventriculostomy in patients with intracranial germinomas. J Neurosurg 2007;107:193–8.

Minimally Invasive Neurosurgery for Vascular Lesions

Nikolai J. Hopf, MD, PhD*, Lars Füllbier, MD

KEYWORDS

- Keyhole craniotomy • Aneurysm surgery • AVM
- Arteriovenous fistula • Cavernoma

Intracranial vascular lesions are known to affect 2% to 4% of the population, predisposing those affected to a lifetime risk of hemorrhagic stroke, ischemia, focal neurologic deficits, or epileptic seizures. These lesions constitute a heterogeneous group, with different lesion types characterized by distinct biologic mechanisms of pathogenesis and progression. In this article, the minimally invasive management of intracranial aneurysms, arteriovenous malformations (AVMs) including arteriovenous fistulas (AVFs), and cavernous malformations are discussed.

ANEURYSMS

The annual incidence of subarachnoid hemorrhage (SAH) from a ruptured intracranial aneurysm in the United States is approximately 1 case per 10,000 persons, yielding approximately 27,000 new cases of SAH each year.[1,2] Autopsy studies indicate a prevalence of intracranial aneurysms of between 1% and 5% in the adult population,[3] which translates to 10 million to 12 million persons in the United States.[1] SAH is more common in women than in men (2:1),[4] and its incidence increases with age, occurring most commonly between 40 and 60 years of age (mean age ≥50 years).[5,6] An estimated 5% to 15% of cases of stroke are related to ruptured intracranial aneurysms.[7]

The most common presentation of intracranial aneurysm is rupture leading to SAH. Given the increased availability of noninvasive imaging techniques, aneurysms are increasingly detected before rupture. An unruptured aneurysm may be asymptomatic and thus be found incidentally, or

it may be diagnosed on the basis of symptoms.[8] Unruptured aneurysms may cause symptoms by exerting mass effect, leading to cranial nerve palsies (eg, the rapid onset of a third nerve palsy caused by the enlargement of an aneurysm of the posterior communicating artery[1]) or brainstem compression.[9] Aneurysms presenting with SAH tend to bleed again. Two percent to four percent of aneurysms hemorrhage again within the first 24 hours after the initial episode, and approximately 15% to 20% bleed a second time within the first 2 weeks.[10,11] Aneurysmal SAH has a 30-day mortality rate of 45%; an estimated 30% of survivors will have moderate to severe disabilities.[12] Aneurysm repair performed after an SAH is generally associated with higher mortality and morbidity rates than elective clipping in unruptured aneurysms.[13] Because of the high risk of rebleeding within the first week, increased treatment risks during the vasospasm period between the 4th and 14th day, and limited medical treatment options for vasospasm in patients with unsecured aneurysms, early treatment (surgical or endovascular) within the first 72 hours following SAH is generally recommended.[13–15] The risk for bleeding in non-ruptured aneurysms depends on aneurysms' size and configuration, localization, and endogenous factors.[16–18] Presently, surgical or endovascular treatment of unruptured aneurysm is recommended in patients having suffered from an SAH caused by another aneurysm and patients bearing symptomatic and/or larger aneurysms (>12 mm). In young patients with positive endogenous factors and/or irregular aneurysm shape, treatment is recommended also in smaller aneurysms.

Department of Neurosurgery, Katharinenhospital, Kriegsbergstrasse 60, Stuttgart D-70174, Germany
* Corresponding author.
E-mail address: n.hopf@klinikum-stuttgart.de

Neurosurg Clin N Am 21 (2010) 673–689
doi:10.1016/j.nec.2010.07.011
1042-3680/10/$ – see front matter © 2010 Elsevier Inc. All rights reserved.

Surgical Treatment

The goal of surgical treatment is to completely exclude the aneurysm from the circulation, without impairment of the cerebral perfusion. This treatment may be enabled by elective clipping or wrapping of the aneurysm or trapping of the affected area of the carrying vessel. The latter may need to be combined with a bypass to maintain sufficient cerebral perfusion. Surgical treatment may also be combined with endovascular techniques, such as stenting and coiling, and may be necessary after technically inadequate endovascular treatment.

Minimally invasive aspects of aneurysm surgery include methods for limiting the exposure of brain tissue using keyhole craniotomies for definitive treatment of ruptured and unruptured aneurysms, reduction of number of required procedures and craniotomies in patients with multiple aneurysms, and reduction of hospitalization time and reconvalescence.

Minimally invasive approaches suitable for aneurysm surgery are the eyebrow, pterional, subtemporal, retrosigmoid, and interhemispheric minicraniotomies (see the article by Garrett and colleagues elsewhere in this issue for further exploration of this topic).

Critical steps involved with the surgical approach to an intracranial aneurysm are sufficient visualization of the associated proximal and distal vessels, early control of the feeding vessel, understanding of the individual pathoanatomy and hemodynamics of the specific aneurysm being treated, dissection of the aneurysm neck, manipulation of the aneurysm dome, selection of appropriate instruments and implants for the definitive treatment, and intraoperative control of the result.

Technical Considerations

Important technical requirements for minimally invasive aneurysm surgery are a high-quality operating microscope that is capable of indocyanine green (ICG) angiography, endoscopes with 0° and 30° viewing angle, and micro-Doppler sonography with 1 and 2 mm probes. In more complex aneurysms, where temporary occlusion or even cardiac arrest is anticipated, neurophysiological monitoring (somatosensory evoked potential [SSEP], motor evoked potential [MEP]) should be performed. Customized clip design and clip appliers are also very helpful to gain sufficient overview in limited craniotomies (**Fig. 1**).

Consideration of all described aspects of minimally invasive aneurysm surgery in combination with proper use of intraoperative modern technology enables successful and safe treatment,

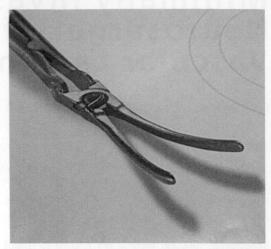

Fig. 1. Special clip applier for limited craniotomies, with fixation of the clip from inside leading to minimal obstruction of the operating field (Peter Lazic, Tuttlingen, Germany; with permission).

with limited exposure in almost all patients with unruptured and ruptured aneurysms.

Specific Surgical Considerations and Illustrative Cases

Anterior circulation aneurysms

The vast majority (90%) of all intracranial aneurysms are located in the anterior circulation, specifically at the anterior communicating artery (AComA) in 30%, the internal carotid artery (ICA) including the posterior communicating artery (PComA) in 30%, and the middle cerebral artery (MCA) in 20%.[11]

The specific challenge for AComA aneurysms is for example the need for control of 2 proximal vessels, that is, the ipsilateral and contralateral A1 segments; for MCA aneurysms it is the high risk of subsequent stroke after temporary occlusion; and for some ICA aneurysms it is the difficulty with obtaining proximal control. However, even complex and large aneurysms may be managed safely through minimally invasive approaches. Preferred approaches for aneurysms of the anterior circulation are the supraorbital keyhole craniotomy (AComA, ICA, MCA), pterional minicraniotomy (ICA, PComA), and the interhemispheric minicraniotomy (pericallosal artery). An example of the technique for minimally invasive management of aneurysms of the anterior circulation is demonstrated in a patient with a previously endovascularly coiled AComA aneurysm.

Case 1: A 52-year-old man suffered from an SAH (Hunt & Hess [H&H] grade I). Angiography revealed an AComA aneurysm (**Fig. 2**A), which was treated by coiling (see **Fig 2**B). A surveillance angiogram 18 months later revealed reopening of

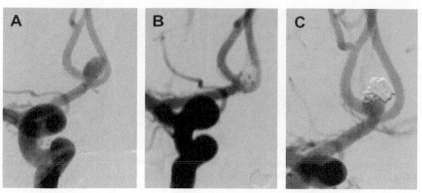

Fig. 2. Cerebral angiography showing the AComA aneurysm (*A*) before and (*B*) after initial complete coiling, (*C*) demonstrating the recanalization in the neck region 18 months later.

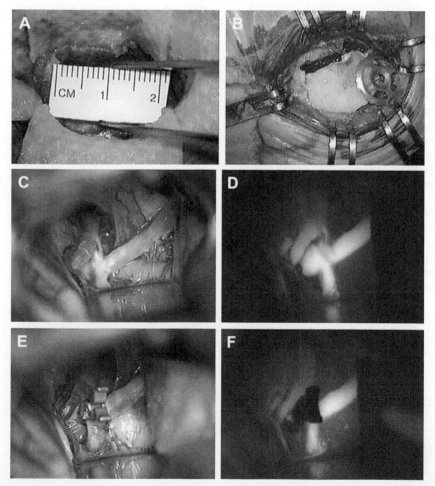

Fig. 3. Intraoperative image of (*A*) the supraorbital keyhole craniotomy before dural opening and (*B*) after reimplantation of the bone flap. Microscopic view of the AComA complex with the aneurysm neck and good overview of both A1 and A2 segments (*C*) before and (*E*) after clipping with the corresponding ICG angiographic images (*D*, *F*).

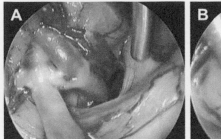

Fig. 4. Different perspective of endoscopic view compared with the microscopic image of the AComA complex demonstrating the aneurysm neck and both A1 and A2 segments (*A*) before and (*B*) after clipping.

the neck (see **Fig. 2**C). Definite surgical treatment was performed through a supraorbital keyhole craniotomy on the right side (**Fig. 3**A and B) using intraoperative ICG angiography (see **Fig. 3**C–F) and endoscope-assisted technique (**Fig. 4**). A postoperative angiogram demonstrated complete aneurysm occlusion (**Fig. 5**).

Posterior circulation aneurysms

Aneurysms of the posterior circulation (basilar artery [BA], posterior cerebral artery [PCA], superior cerebellar artery [SCA], vertebral artery [VA], posterior inferior cerebellar artery [PICA]) represent only about 10% of intracranial aneurysms.[11] Most of these aneurysms are presently managed using endovascular techniques because of the high rate of morbidity associated with transcranial surgical approaches. However, unfavorable anatomy of the aneurysm or alterations in the proximal vessel may still mandate surgical management. Preferred minimally invasive approaches to the posterior circulation are the supraorbital keyhole craniotomy (BA, PCA, SCA), the subtemporal minicraniotomy (BA, PCA, SCA), and the retrosigmoid minicraniotomy (PICA, VA). Minimally invasive management of aneurysms of the posterior

circulation is demonstrated in a patient with a pre-treated formerly ruptured PICA aneurysm.

Case 2: A 58-year-old woman suffered from an SAH from a ruptured PICA aneurysm. This hemorrhage was initially treated by endovascular coiling. A routine angiogram demonstrated significant recanalization of the neck (**Fig. 6**). Surgical clipping via a retrosigmoid minicraniotomy was performed. Endoscope-assisted technique was used to enhance understanding of the aneurysm pathoanatomy before and after clipping (**Fig. 7**). Despite this complex clinical situation, complete occlusion of the aneurysm was achieved through a limited approach (**Fig. 8**).

Multiple aneurysms

More than 1 aneurysm is found in 10% to 30% of all patients with aneurysm.[1] Aneurysm distribution

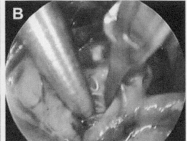

Fig. 5. Postoperative cerebral angiography showing the complete occlusion of the AComA aneurysm (*A*) with and (*B*) without subtraction.

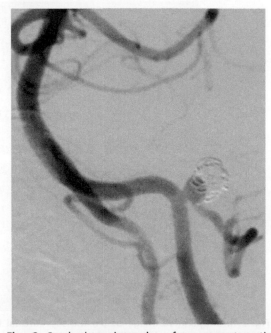

Fig. 6. Cerebral angiography of an asymptomatic patient with a history of SAH and endovascular coiling of a left-sided PICA aneurysm showing recanalization.

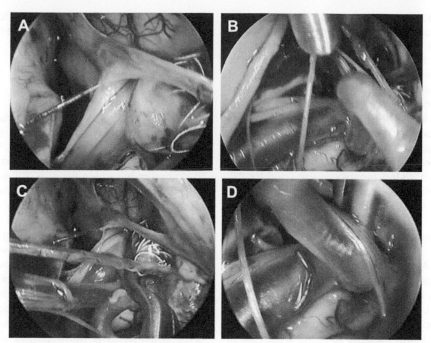

Fig. 7. Intraoperative endoscopic image of the PICA aneurysm in the left cerebellopontine angle, (*A*) demonstrating the proximal and lateral aspects of the neck, (*B*) close-up of the PICA, (*C*) overview after clipping, and (*D*) close-up showing the uncompromised PICA.

in these patients follows the same patterns as seen in patients with single aneurysms. Basically, all potential combinations of multiple aneurysms can be seen. The minimally invasive surgical strategy for addressing multiple aneurysms is to occlude as many aneurysms as possible through a single craniotomy, which means that sometimes not all aneurysms can be addressed via the optimal approach.[19] A thorough analysis of possible approaches to each aneurysm and possible additional risks associated with applying this strategy is mandatory to struggle for the best treatment of any individual patient. Preferred approaches for multiple aneurysms are the supraorbital keyhole craniotomy and the pterional minicraniotomy. Minimally invasive management of multiple aneurysms is demonstrated in a patient with incidental bilateral MCA aneurysms and a patient with a ruptured BA aneurysm and an unruptured right ICA aneurysm.

Case 3: A 58-year-old woman was referred with an H&H grade IV SAH and atypical right frontal intracerebral hemorrhage (ICH). Angiography revealed multiple aneurysms of both MCA and the

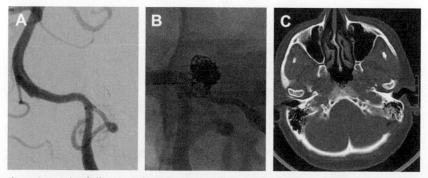

Fig. 8. Cerebral angiography following clipping, (*A*) with and (*B*) without subtraction showing perfect reconstruction of the PICA, clip location, and the coils left inside; (*C*) postoperative computed tomography showing the retromastoid minicraniectomy.

right ICA. Based on the location of the ICH, the right ICA aneurysm was thought to be the bleeding source. Coil occlusion of the ICA aneurysm was performed. Surveillance angiography 6 months later demonstrated complete coil occlusion of the ICA aneurysm, but 4 additional aneurysms were located at the right M1, right ICA bifurcation, left M1, and left M2 (**Fig. 9**). The patient had recovered well from her hemorrhage and therefore was offered surgical occlusion of all further aneurysms via a unilateral supraorbital keyhole craniotomy. Endoscope-assisted technique was used for the ipsilateral (**Fig. 10**) and the contralateral aneurysms (**Fig. 11**). Complete occlusion of all aneurysms was achieved without complications as demonstrated by postoperative angiography (**Fig. 12**).

Case 4: A 68-year-old woman suffered from acute headache and dizziness. A computed tomography of the head showed a basal and right sylvian SAH. Angiography revealed an aneurysm of the BA tip, thought to be the bleeding source, and an incidental medially directed aneurysm of the right proximal ICA (**Fig. 13**). Endovascular treatment was felt to be a poor option because of severe arteriosclerotic changes of the VAs and BA, and a rather broad neck of the BA aneurysm. Occlusion of both aneurysms was achieved using a left supraorbital keyhole craniotomy. Endoscope-assisted technique was used to enhance the understanding the pathoanatomy of the basilar tip aneurysm before and after clipping (**Fig. 14**). The contralateral location of the craniotomy to the right ICA aneurysm was chosen because of the medial orientation of the aneurysm, which could be visualized well from the opposite side using the endoscope (**Fig. 15**). Postoperative angiography demonstrated complete occlusion of both aneurysms (**Fig. 16**).

SUMMARY

Today, ruptured and unruptured aneurysms of all locations may be surgically treated successfully using minimally invasive techniques. In choosing the correct keyhole approach, it becomes possible to dramatically reduce the size of the craniotomy with less brain exposure and retraction, thereby minimizing clipping-related morbidity.[19] Minimally invasive surgical management of aneurysms provides the possibility of enabling the higher long-term occlusion rates possible with surgical management, with a more favorable morbidity profile. By diminishing the risk profile of open surgery, coupled with the benefits of less frequent and less invasive follow-up investigations, the microsurgical management of aneurysms may once again become the treatment of choice for patients with ruptured and unruptured aneurysms. However, minimally invasive aneurysm surgery requires thorough planning, a strong commitment of the surgical team to improving their technique with these methods, the availability of modern technical equipment, and a comprehensive knowledge of neurovascular pathoanatomy and pathophysiology. Therefore, minimally invasive aneurysm surgery should be performed preferably in high-volume and specialized neurovascular centers, which continuously monitor and assess their results with the goal of continuously improving their treatment protocols.

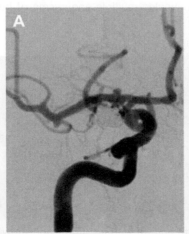 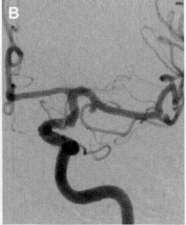

Fig. 9. Cerebral angiography of (*A*) the coil-occluded right ICA aneurysm and 2 further small aneurysms of the right M1 and right ICA bifurcation, (*B*) left ICA with further 2 small aneurysms of the M1 and M2 segments.

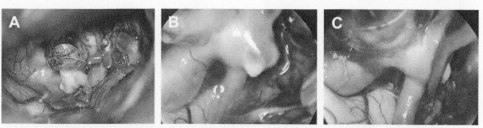

Fig. 10. (*A–C*) Intraoperative microscopic image showing the right coil-occluded ICA aneurysm, the clipped right M1 aneurysm, and the additional aneurysm of the ICA bifurcation; endoscopic view of the aneurysm of the right ICA bifurcation (*A*) before and (*C*) after clipping with perfect view of the large perforator.

ARTERIOVENOUS MALFORMATIONS

Cerebral AVMs are congenital vascular malformations consisting of a network of feeding arteries and draining veins within the brain parenchyma, in which loss of normal vascular organization at the subarteriolar level without an intervening capillary bed results in abnormal arteriovenous shunting. The direct arteriovenous connection leads to fibromuscular thickening and incompetent elastica interna particularly in veins, with an increased risk of rupture.[20] Malformations with only 1 feeding vessel that lack an intervening nidus

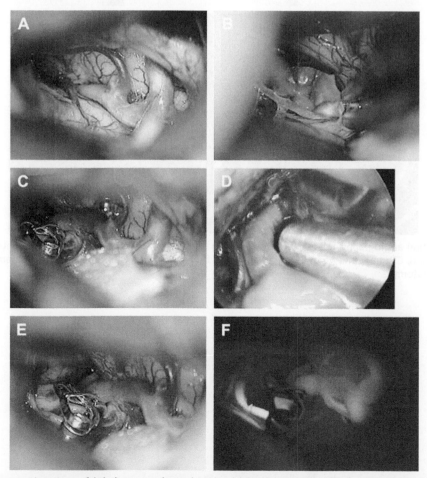

Fig. 11. Intraoperative view of (*A*) the contralateral M1 and (*B*) M2 aneurysm, (*C*) showing both aneurysms clipped with the non-involved M2 segment running through the clip fenestration, (*D*) endoscopic clip control showing the involved M2 without compression, (*E*) microscopic image and (*F*) ICG angiography of the clipped contralateral M2 aneurysm.

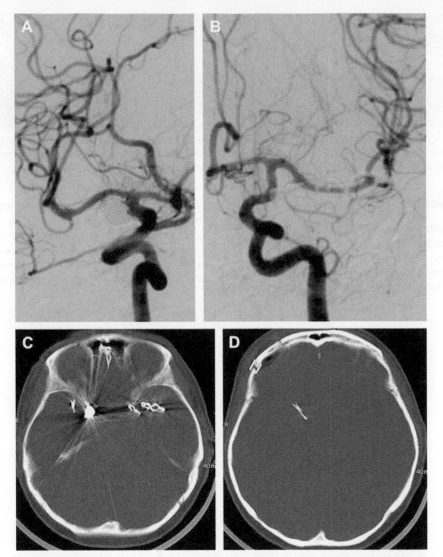

Fig. 12. Cerebral angiography following clipping of (A) all ipsilateral right-sided and (B) all contralateral left-sided aneurysms; CT image showing (C) all clips inserted from the right side and (D) the right-sided supraorbital keyhole craniotomy.

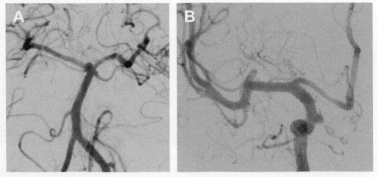

Fig. 13. Cerebral angiography of a patient presenting with an SAH from (A) a BA tip aneurysm and (B) an additional incidental right ICA aneurysm.

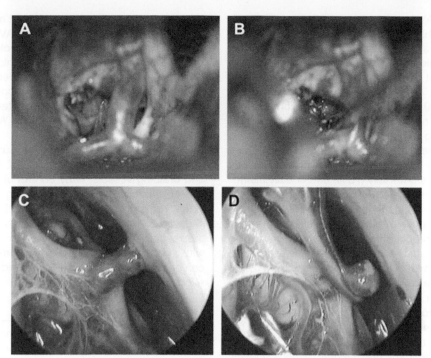

Fig. 14. Intraoperative microscopic view via a left supraorbital keyhole craniotomy of the posterior cerebral artery and the basilar artery tip aneurysm (*A*) before and (*B*) during clipping. Endoscopic view of the same aneurysm (*C*) before and (*D*) after clipping.

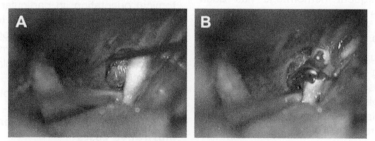

Fig. 15. Intraoperative microscopic view of the additional incidental right ICA aneurysm (*A*) before and (*B*) after clipping.

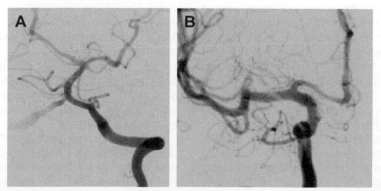

Fig. 16. Cerebral angiography after endoscope-assisted clip occlusion of (*A*) the BA tip aneurysm and (*B*) the incidental right ICA aneurysm via a left supraorbital keyhole craniotomy.

are called AVFs. If the location of the fistula is located within the dura, they are called dural AVFs (DAVFs). DAVFs are thought to be acquired.

The prevalence of arteriovenous malformation is estimated at approximately 0.1% of the general population, but reported rates range from 0.001% to 0.52%.[20] AVMs may become symptomatic by rupture, leading to ICH and/or SAH but can also cause symptoms without rupturing by causing seizures, symptoms due to mass effect, or ischemic steal. AVMs are most commonly located supratentorially (75%) and equally distributed within the cerebral lobes. AVMs occur less frequently in the insula and basal ganglia.

The overall risk of hemorrhage of arteriovenous malformations is estimated to range from 2% to 4% per year, and each hemorrhage is associated with a 5% to 10% chance of death and a 30% to 50% chance of permanent, disabling neurologic deficits.[20] In most patients, the first hemorrhage typically occurs between 20 and 40 years of age.[20,21] The risk of bleeding is increased by the presence of aneurysms (feeding artery, intranidal, or venous), drainage into the deep venous sinuses, deep location (ie, basal ganglia, internal capsule, thalamus, or corpus callosum), a single draining vein, venous stenosis, and previous hemorrhage.[20,22–24] After first hemorrhage, the annual risk of a subsequent hemorrhage has been reported to range from 4.5% to 34.4% during the first year, with a return to the baseline risk after the first year.[20,23]

Immediate surgical treatment is indicated only in space occupying ICH. Preoperative embolization may be helpful also in these cases. Contemporary treatment strategies include in most instances an initial endovascular embolization, often in a multi-step procedure, followed by surgical resection or radiosurgery.

Surgical Treatment

The goal of surgical treatment is to completely occlude or resect the nidus or fistula without impairment of the normal cerebral perfusion. Partial occlusion or resection of the AVM does not lead to a relevant reduction of the bleeding risk. The risk of treatment in AVMs can be estimated by the Spetzler-Martin grading system. Larger size (<3, 3–6, >6 cm), eloquent location, and deep venous drainage were found to be associated with a higher treatment risk.[25]

Minimally invasive aspects of AVM surgery involve limiting the exposure for complete occlusion or resection of the AVM or AVF and highly selective occlusion or resection of ill-defined vessels, thereby leading to reduction of hospitalization time and reconvalescence.

Basically, all previously mentioned minimally invasive approaches are suitable for AVM and AVF surgery, that is, the supraorbital keyhole, pterional, retrosigmoid, and interhemispheric minicraniotomies (see the article by Garrett and colleagues elsewhere in this issue for further exploration of this topic). But frequently an individually tailored craniotomy has to be placed over the AVM on the convexity of the skull.

Critical aspects for successful surgical treatment are sufficient visualization of the feeding and draining vessels, early control of the feeding vessel, intraoperative understanding of the individual haemodynamics, proper occlusion of the ill-defined vessels, and intraoperative control of the result. Applying this concept in combination with modern technology, even complex AVMs can be successfully and safely treated with limited exposure.

Technical Considerations

Necessary requirements for minimally invasive AVM surgery is a high-quality operating microscope equipped with ICG angiography. Alternatively, high-quality sonography or micro-Doppler sonography may be used intraoperatively to assess the individual haemodynamics. Endoscopes may also be helpful to enhance pathoanatomical orientation, in particular in DAVFs. In all AVMs with relevant relation to the motor or sensory cortex neurophysiological monitoring (SSEP, MEP) should be performed. Occlusion of the AVM is performed by bipolar coagulation or application of clips. Specific nonstick bipolar coagulation forceps are advisable.

Specific Surgical Considerations and Illustrative Cases

The surgical strategy is to secure early control of all feeding vessels while carefully sparing the draining veins. At the end of the resection, the veins should be occluded or resected if not involved in important drainage of healthy brain tissue to avoid recruitment of new arterial vessels and thus leading to recurrence. Furthermore, the complete nidus should be removed, even the embolized parts. Minimally invasive management of AVMs is demonstrated in a patient with a left-sided parieto-occipital AVM and a patient with an ethmoidal DAVF.

Case 5: A 19-year-old boy suffered from a left-sided atypical ICH. Angiography revealed a left occipital grade III (Spetzler-Martin) AVM (**Fig. 17**). Partial embolization was achieved leaving still a multicompartmental AVM with significant arteriovenous shunt. At that time, the patient had visual

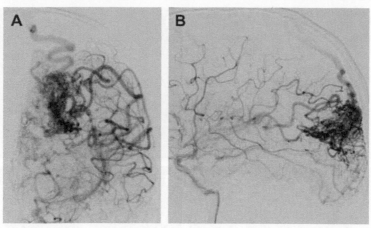

Fig. 17. Cerebral angiography of a left occipital AVM in (*A*) anteroposterior and (*B*) lateral views.

field deficits at the lower right quadrant. Complete surgical resection was performed through a tailored paramedian parieto-occipital craniotomy in prone position with the aid of neuronavigation and intraoperative ICG angiography (**Fig. 18**).

Case 6: In a 69-year-old man who suffered from an SAH 15 years ago, angiography at that time did not show a bleeding source. A ventriculoperitoneal shunt had to be inserted because of posthemorrhagic hydrocephalus. Now, a follow-up magnetic resonance imaging (MRI) revealed a significant stenosis of the right MCA. Angiography showed complete occlusion of the right MCA but sufficient perfusion of the right hemisphere. In addition, it revealed a left-sided ethmoidal DAVF at the basal and frontal aspects of the falx (**Fig. 19**A). An endovascular treatment trial was unsuccessful. Complete surgical occlusion was achieved using an endoscope-assisted technique (see **Fig. 19**B; **Fig. 20**A) through a left-sided supraorbital keyhole craniotomy using intraoperative ICG angiography (see **Fig. 20**C–F).

SUMMARY

Contemporary treatment of AVMs involves a team approach among neuroradiologists, neurosurgeons, and radiation oncologists. Initial embolization reduces surgical morbidity, blood loss, and operating time. Generally, complete destruction by resection or irradiation is required to cure the disease. AVMs frequently involve larger areas of the brain surface. Therefore, limited craniotomies are often not applicable. However, when possible, minimally invasive approaches to the treatment of AVMs consist of a tailored craniotomy, strict intraoperative strategic workflow, and advanced intraoperative visualization and resection control using ICG angiography and/or technologically advanced sonography. As with all minimally invasive neurosurgical procedures, AVM surgery requires thorough planning, an organized team dedicated to neuroendoscopy, availability of modern technical equipment, and an extraordinary knowledge of neurovascular pathoanatomy and pathophysiology. Treatment of AVMs should be performed in experienced centers that are capable of performing all available treatment modalities (ie, endovascular, surgical, and radiation therapies).

CAVERNOUS MALFORMATIONS (CAVERNOMAS)

Cavernous malformations (cavernomas) are benign vascular lesions consisting of cavernous-like enlarged veins with dysplastic walls located within the brain or rarely in the spinal cord lacking intervening neural parenchyma, large feeding arteries, or large draining veins.[26,27] Cavernomas affect 0.4% to 0.5% of the population[27] and become symptomatic either by bleeding (20%) and thereby leading to an (often small) ICH with headaches and/or focal neurologic deficits, or frequently by initiating epileptic seizures (60%).[27,28] Most of all cavernomas are located supratentorially, but 10% to 23% are found in the brainstem, the cerebellum, and the myelon. Within the brainstem, there is a predilection for formation in the pons.[27] Two-thirds of the spinal cavernomas are located in the thoracic and one-third in the cervical myelon. In 15% of all cases, cavernomas are associated with a so-called developmental venous anomaly. The bleeding rate is variable and the definition of symptomatic hemorrhage is controversial; however, the overall

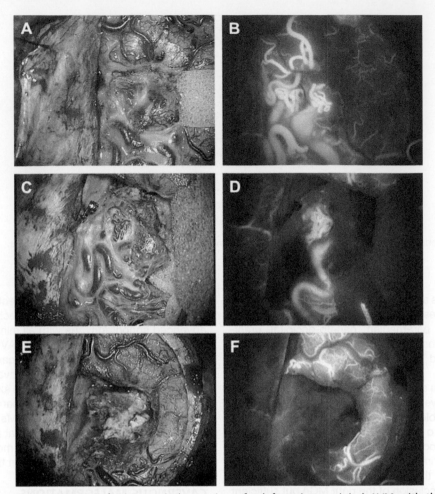

Fig. 18. Intraoperative images of microsurgical resection of a left parieto-occipital AVM with the patient in a prone position, (*A*) before, (*C*) after occlusion of the medial compartment of the AVM, and (*E*) after complete resection with the corresponding images of the intraoperative ICG angiography (*B, D, F*). The medial vein seems to be still arterialized as seen under the microscope (*C*), but ICG angiography (*D*) clearly shows no arteriovenous shunt anymore in that compartment of the AVM.

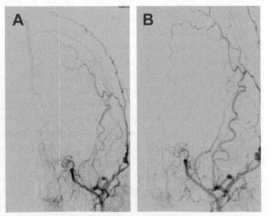

Fig. 19. Cerebral angiography of the left external carotid artery showing (*A*) a left fronto-mediobasal (ethmoidal) DAVF, (*B*) postopertively in coronal view.

rate is estimated between 0.6% and 3.1% per year.[27,28] Cavernomas situated in the brainstem or the cerebellum tend to bleed more easily and cause more damage than those found in the cerebrum.

Surgical Treatment

The goal of surgical treatment is to completely resect the cavernoma. In patients with seizures and supratentorially located lesions, removal of the surrounding yellowish gliosis harboring epileptogenic ferritin deposits should be addressed if not located in a highly eloquent region. The only effective treatment for cavernomas is complete surgical resection. Radiotherapy including radiosurgery has not conclusively been demonstrated to alter the natural history of these lesions.

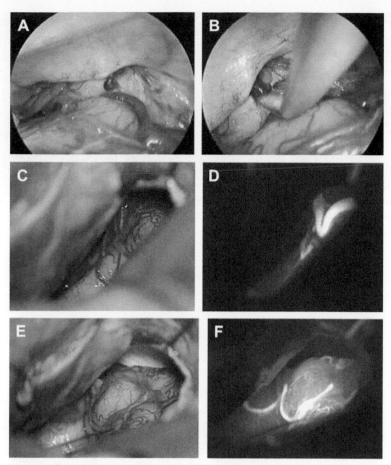

Fig. 20. Endoscopic view of a left fronto-medio-basal DAVF approached via a left supraorbital keyhole craniotomy (*A*) before and (*B*) during treatment. Microscopic and ICG angiographic images (*C, D*) before and (*E, F*) after coagulation and transsection of the DAVF.

Minimally invasive aspects of cavernoma surgery involve reduction of approach-related morbidity in deep-seated and brainstem lesions, lesionectomy-related morbidity, and hospitalization and back-to-work time. Minimally invasive approaches suitable for brainstem cavernomas are the eyebrow, pterional, subtemporal, retrosigmoid, and suboccipital minicraniotomies (see the article by Garrett and colleagues elsewhere in this issue for further exploration of this topic).

Critical aspects for successful surgical treatment are selection of the optimal approach, improved intraoperative visualization by using an endoscope, recognition of fiber tracks and anatomic landmarks using neuronavigation, electrophysiological monitoring of fiber tracks and cranial nerve nuclei, selection of microsurgical instruments suitable for complete removal of the lesion, and intraoperative control of the result, namely obtaining adequate hemostasis following lesionectomy. Applying

this concept in combination with advanced technology, most deep-seated and even brainstem cavernomas can be successfully and safely removed.

Technical Considerations

The basic requirements for minimally invasive cavernoma surgery are a high-quality operating microscope and a neuronavigation system. Alternatively, high-quality sonography may be used intraoperatively to visualize a deep-seated cavernoma. Endoscopes may also be helpful to enhance pathoanatomic orientation, in particular to screen for remnants in the resection cavity. Detailed neurophysiological monitoring (concentric needle electromyography/stimulation, SSEP, MEP, auditory evoked potential) is mandatory in all brainstem cavernomas and other highly eloquent locations.

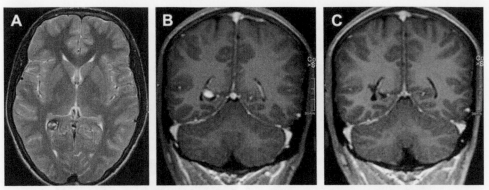

Fig. 21. (*A*) T2-weighted axial and (*B*) T1-weighted coronal gadolinium-enhanced MRI of a right temporo-occipital deep-seated cavernoma (*B*) before and (*C*) after complete removal.

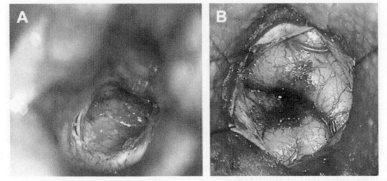

Fig. 22. Microscopic view (*A*) through the right lateral ventricle into the resection cavity after complete removal of the cavernoma and (*B*) of the transsulcal, transcortical approach at the end of the surgery.

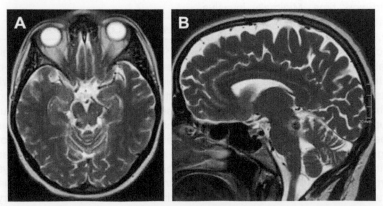

Fig. 23. T2-weighted (*A*) axial and (*B*) sagittal MRI of a patient with a right dorsolateral cavernoma of the midbrain.

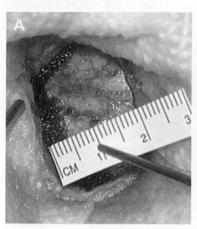
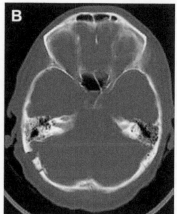

Fig. 24. Right-sided osteoplastic retrosigmoid minicraniotomy (*A*) before opening of the dura and (*B*) in the computed tomographic scan postoperatively, the bone flap fixed with CranioFix (B.Braun/Aesculap, Tuttlingen, Germany; with permission).

Specific Surgical Considerations and Illustrative Cases

It is critical to approach the cavernoma in the least traumatic manner. Compared with other neurovascular lesions, dealing with the lesion itself is often less difficult than approaching the lesion, which is particularly true in the case of deep-seated and brainstem cavernomas. As a rule of thumb, a cavernoma is best approached from where it reaches any surface of the brain. In some cases, this region may be the ependymal surface of the ventricular system.

The cases below demonstrate minimally invasive management of cavernomas in a patient with a deep-seated cavernoma of the right temporo-occipital paraventricular region and a patient with a symptomatic brainstem cavernoma.

Case 7: A 15-year-old boy presented with severe headaches but otherwise neurologically intact. MRI showed a right temporo-occipital paraventricular lesion, typical for a cavernoma (**Fig. 21**A, B). A transtemporal, transventricular minimally invasive approach (**Fig. 22**) was used for complete removal (see **Fig. 21**C). With the aid of neuronavigation, the optic fibers could be spared. Postoperatively, the patient was completely neurologically intact, in particular with no visual field deficits.

Case 8: A 48-year-old woman suddenly developed numbness and sensory deficits of the right side of her body. MRI showed a cavernoma of the right dorsolateral midbrain (**Fig. 23**). A right-sided retromastoid (**Fig. 24**), supracerebellar keyhole approach was chosen for complete removal (**Fig. 25**) with the support of neuronavigation, endoscopy, and, neurophysiological monitoring.

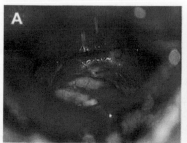
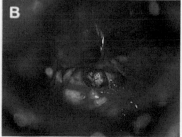

Fig. 25. Intraoperative microscopic view of the dorsolateral midbrain showing (*A*) the yellowish discoloration from the cavernoma bleeding and (*B*) the empty cavity after complete removal.

SUMMARY

Cavernomas are frequently found in highly eloquent and/or deep locations. Complete surgical removal is the only proven treatment for definitive management of these lesions. Surgical morbidity is not only related to the lesionectomy but also to the approach. Minimally invasive concepts may help to reduce both approach-related and lesionectomy-related morbidities. Thorough planning and the willingness to familiarize oneself with these challenging and often unfamiliar approaches is an essential requirement for safe and technically successful minimally invasive cavernoma surgery. Furthermore, technical preconditions such as advanced neuronavigation and multimodal neurophysiological monitoring are essential for clinical success.

REFERENCES

1. Schievink WI. Intracranial aneurysms. N Engl J Med 1997;336:28–40 [erratum in: N Engl J Med 1997; 336:1267].

2. Wijdicks EF, Kallmes DF, Manno EM, et al. Subarachnoid hemorrhage: neurointensive care and aneurysm repair. Mayo Clin Proc 2005;80:550–9.

3. Wiebers DO, Whisnant JP, Huston J III, et al. Unruptured intracranial aneurysms: natural history, clinical outcome, and risks of surgical and endovascular treatment. Lancet 2003;362:103–10.

4. Stapf C, Mohr JP. Aneurysms and subarachnoid hemorrhage epidemiology. In: Le Roux PD, Winn HR, Newell DW, editors. Management of cerebral aneurysms. Philadelphia: Saunders; 2004. p. 183–7.

5. Rinkel GJ, Djibuti M, Algra A, et al. Prevalence and risk of rupture of intracranial aneurysms: a systematic review. Stroke 1998;29:251–6.

6. Bederson JB, Connolly ES, Batjer HH, et al. Guidelines for the management of aneurismal subarachnoid hemorrhage. A statement for the healthcare professionals from a special writing group of the stroke council, American Heart Association. Stroke 2009;40:994–1025.

7. Bederson JB, Awad IA, Wiebers DO, et al. Recommendations for the management of patients with unruptured intracranial aneurysms: a statement for healthcare professionals from the stroke council of the American Heart Association. Stroke 2000;31: 2742–50.

8. Suarez JI, Tarr RW, Selman WR. Aneurysmal subarachnoid hemorrhage. N Engl J Med 2006; 354:387–96.

9. Connolly ES, Solomon RA. Management of unruptured aneurysms. In: Le Roux PD, Winn HR, Newell DW, editors. Management of cerebral aneurysms. Philadelphia: Saunders; 2004. p. 271–85.

10. Greenberg MS. SAH and aneurysms. In: Greenberg MS, editor. Handbook of neurosurgery. 5th edition. New York: Thieme Medical; 2000. p. 754–803.

11. Brisman JL, Song JK, Newell DW. Cerebral aneurysms. N Engl J Med 2006;355:928–39.

12. Johnston SC, Selvin S, Gress DR. The burden, trends, and demographics of mortality from subarachnoid hemorrhage. Neurology 1998;50:1413–8.

13. Raaymakers TWM, Rinkle GJ, Limburg M, et al. Mortality and morbidity of surgery for unruptured intracranial aneurysms: a meta-analysis. Stroke 1998;29:1531–8.

14. Hunt WE, Hess RM. Surgical risk as related to time of intervention in the repair of intracranial aneurysms. J Neurosurg 1968;28(1):14–20.

15. Whitfield PC, Kirkpatrick PJ. Timing of surgery for aneurysmal subarachnoid hemorrhage. Cochrane Database Syst Rev 2001;2:CD001697.

16. International Study of Unruptured Intracranial Aneurysms Investigators (ISUIA). Unruptured intracranial aneurysms – risk of rupture and risk of surgical intervention. N Engl J Med 1998;339:1725–33.

17. Clarke G, Mendelow AD, Mitchell P. Predicting the risk of rupture of intracranial aneurysms based on anatomical location. Acta Neurochir 2005;147: 259–63.

18. International Study of Unruptured Intracranial Aneurysms Investigators (ISUIA). Unruptured intracranial aneurysms: natural history, clinical outcome, and risks of surgical and endovascular treatment. Lancet 2003;362:103–10.

19. Hopf NJ, Stadie A, Reisch R. Surgical management of bilateral middle cerebral artery aneurysms via a unilateral supraorbital key-hole craniotomy. Minim Invasive Neurosurg 2009;52:126–31.

20. Friedlander RM. Arteriovenous malformations of the brain. N Engl J Med 2007;356(26):2704–12.

21. Brown RD Jr, Wiebers DO, Torner JC, et al. Frequency of intracranial hemorrhage as a presenting symptom and subtype analysis: a population-based study of intracranial vascular malformations in Olmsted Country, Minnesota. J Neurosurg 1996; 85:29–32.

22. Redekop G, TerBrugge K, Montanera W, et al. Arterial aneurysms associated with cerebral arteriovenous malformations: classification, incidence, and risk of hemorrhage. J Neurosurg 1998;89:539–46.

23. Stapf C, Mast H, Sciacca RR, et al. Predictors of hemorrhage in patients with untreated brain arteriovenous malformation. Neurology 2006;66:1350–5.

24. Nataf F, Meder JF, Roux FX. Angioarchitecture associated with hemorrhage in cerebral arteriovenous malformations: a prognostic statistical model. Neuroradiology 1997;39:52–8.

25. Spetzler RF, Martin NA. A proposed grading system for arteriovenous malformations 1986. J Neurosurg 2008;65:476–83.

26. Robinson JR, Awad IA, Little JR. Natural history of the cavernous angioma. J Neurosurg 1991;75:709–14.

27. Greenberg MS. Handbook of neurosurgery. 6th edition. New York: Thieme Medical Publishers; 2006.

28. Amin-Hanjani S, Ojemann RG, Ogilvy CS. Surgical management of cavernous malformations of the nervous system. In: Roberts DW, Schmidek HH, editors. Schmidek & sweet's operative neurosurgical techniques. indications, methods, and results. 5th edition. Philadelphia: Saunders Elsevier; 2006. p. 1307–24.

Minimally Invasive Surgery for Movement Disorders

Paul S. Larson, MD[a,b],*

KEYWORDS

- Deep brain stimulation • Stereotactic surgery
- Frameless deep brain stimulation • Interventional MRI
- Gene transfer

Surgery for movement disorders has become commonplace over the last decade, and is now considered the standard of care for properly selected candidates with moderately advanced, medically refractory disease. Although many movement disorders have been treated with surgery over the course of the last century including tremor and dystonia, by far the most common indication for surgery today is Parkinson disease (PD). Likewise, there have been several different procedures used, including open craniotomy and stereotactic lesioning, in several different brain targets in the cortical and subcortical regions. In the modern era, deep brain stimulation (DBS) is the procedure of choice. Unlike lesioning procedures, which result in permanent destruction of the brain, DBS provides adjustable and reversible modulation of brain function, thus affording clinicians the opportunity to maximize benefits while minimizing side effects of stimulation. When considering minimally invasive surgical strategies for movement disorders, it is therefore helpful to use DBS for PD as a model; it is the most frequently performed procedure in movement disorders surgery, and many of the principles used in DBS for PD are applicable to other stereotactic procedures.

In comparison with other topics discussed in this book, DBS would already be considered by many to be a minimally invasive procedure. DBS is traditionally performed through a single burr hole with the use of a stereotactic frame; most patients with PD gain the most benefit with bilateral electrode implantation, so patients receive 2 burr holes (approximately 14–15 mm in diameter) through 1 longer or 2 smaller incisions. At present, the most commonly implanted target for DBS implantation in PD is the subthalamic nucleus (STN), although stimulation of the globus pallidus internus (GPi) is equally effective in treating the cardinal symptoms of PD, and parkinsonian tremor in isolation can be treated with stimulation of the thalamus. All of these targets are relatively deep in the subcortex, with the STN being the deepest. As a result, one must choose a trajectory through the brain that causes minimal potential injury and would result in the least amount of morbidity if a hemorrhage were to occur during electrode placement. Virtually all centers place the burr hole at or just anterior to the coronal suture, which provides a trajectory through noneloquent frontal cortex in which a hemorrhage would be well tolerated.

In general, the goals for a minimally invasive approach to DBS would decrease patient discomfort, reduce operative time, and/or minimize penetration of the brain. When contemplating how to approach DBS for PD from a minimally invasive

This article describes work that was supported by research grants and support to the author from Medtronic, Inc, Surgivision, Inc, Ceregene, Inc, and Genzyme, Inc.

[a] Department of Neurological Surgery, University of California, San Francisco, 505 Parnassus Avenue, Box 0112, San Francisco, CA 94143-0112, USA

[b] San Francisco VA Medical Center, 4150 Clement Street, PADRECC 127P, San Francisco, CA 94121, USA

* Department of Neurological Surgery, University of California, San Francisco, 505 Parnassus Avenue, Box 0112, San Francisco, CA 94143-0112.

E-mail address: larsonp@neurosurg.ucsf.edu

Neurosurg Clin N Am 21 (2010) 691–698
doi:10.1016/j.nec.2010.07.012
1042-3680/10/$ – see front matter. Published by Elsevier Inc.

perspective, one must accept that the entry point, trajectory, targets, and number of electrodes are relatively inflexible given the knowledge of the brain nuclei involved in PD and the basic principles of safe stereotactic surgery. The variable factors are (1) the delivery device, that is, the device used to place the electrode into the brain, (2) the target localization method, that is, the method used by the surgeon to make sure the electrode is going to the desired target in the brain, and (3) the hardware used to modulate the desired target in the brain. The method by which these variables can be manipulated to provide more minimally invasive methodologies for DBS surgery is examined here. It should be mentioned that these methods could be applied to other stereotactic procedures including lesioning, cannula-based infusions, biopsy, and so forth.

DELIVERY DEVICE

The traditional delivery devices in DBS surgery are a stereotactic frame and a micropositioner that allows precise, mechanical manipulation of both micro- and macroelectrodes during surgery (**Fig. 1**). A variety of frames are available from several major manufacturers including the Leksell (Elekta, Stockholm, Sweden) and CRW (Integra Radionics, Burlington, MA, USA) frames. Most centers that perform DBS use a stereotactic frame with some combination of magnetic resonance imaging (MRI) and computed tomography (CT), and a surgical planning workstation such as the StealthStation (Medtronic, Minneapolis, MN). Although frame-based implantation has a long record of safety and tolerability and remains the most common delivery method for DBS, in the last decade many surgeons have

started to adopt so-called frameless techniques, which include use of the commercially available STarFix micro Targeting Platform (FHC, Bowdoinham, ME, USA) and the Nexframe (Medtronic, Minneapolis, MN, USA). The move toward frameless techniques was motivated in part by trying to apply some of the principles of minimally invasive surgery to DBS. In this instance, the variable that was modified was the delivery device, and the goals were to decrease patient discomfort and reduce operative time.

Both the STarFix and Nexframe use bone-implanted fiducial markers, which are significantly more stable and reliable than skin-based fiducials. Such markers allow these platforms to equal the application accuracy of traditional stereotactic frames, which makes frameless DBS a legitimate alternative.[1] Proponents of frameless DBS claim that insertion of the bone-implanted fiducials is more comfortable than application of a stereotactic frame. Moreover, the patients are not rigidly fixed to the operating table as they are when they are in a frame, which allows them to change position slightly during surgery if desired. Perhaps most significant, however, is that the bone-implanted fiducials can be inserted days or even weeks before surgery, meaning that the preoperative imaging, targeting, and planning can all be done before the day of the procedure. This scheduling radically streamlines the patient flow on the day of surgery; the patient can go straight to the operating room instead of having to undergo frame placement, followed by imaging, and then waiting while the surgeon performs targeting and trajectory planning before starting the case. For patients with PD, who are typically kept off parkinsonian medications on the day of surgery to optimize the process of physiologic mapping and avoid dyskinesias, this can be of great advantage. One of the significant sources of patient discomfort during DBS surgery for PD is being in the off-medication state, and anything that reduces the procedure time usually translates to less discomfort for the patient.

Beyond the shared use of bone-implanted fiducials, the STarFix and Nexframe techniques diverge significantly. In the STarFix platform, the bone-implanted fiducials are used not as a basis for optical tracking, but rather as markers to define the geometry of a custom-made, patient-specific, skull-mounted aiming device. Days or even weeks before surgery, the surgeon implants the bone markers in a specified manner around the typical entry point in the frontal region and obtains high-resolution CT and MRI. Target selection, trajectory planning, and burr hole location are all determined within a proprietary software program; when the

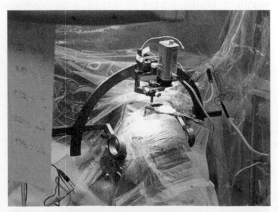

Fig. 1. A typical stereotactic frame and micropositioner system being used intraoperatively for performing multichannel microelectrode recording and DBS electrode placement.

surgeon is done, the software generates a blueprint for the STarFix platform. This disposable platform consists of a small ring (which ultimately holds a multilumen insert through which guide tubes and electrodes can be passed), and 3 or 4 legs that angle downward and are designed to anchor to the skull via the previously implanted bone fiducials. Every platform blueprint that the software creates is unique and based on the location of the bone markers as well as the entry point, trajectory, and target as determined by the surgeon. Platforms for unilateral or simultaneous bilateral implants can be created.

Once the surgeon is satisfied, the blueprint is electronically sent to a manufacturing center in which the platform is made using rapid prototyping technologies, then shipped back to the implanting hospital. The platform is sterilized and attached to the bone-implanted markers during surgery, which have been left in the skull during the intervening period between target imaging and surgery. The platform can be attached and removed at will, giving the surgeon free access to the head for opening and burr hole formation. During actual electrode implantation, the platform allows the surgeon to use standard target localization methods including single or multichannel microelectrode recording (MER). Other advantages unique to this frameless system include relatively free access to the burr hole for anchoring the electrode and the freedom from relying on optical tracking devices for registration, which can be a time-consuming and sometimes finicky process. One disadvantage of the STarFix is the relative inflexibility in the trajectory and burr hole site once the platform is manufactured.

The Nexframe is the other commercially available frameless delivery device. Nowadays it is much more widely used than the STarFix, and the way it works is much more familiar to surgeons who use neuronavigation for other cranial and spinal procedures. The Nexframe uses fiducial-based optical tracking technology, with the bone-implanted fiducials in this instance acting truly as markers only; the actual aiming device is mounted directly to the skull around the burr hole with self-tapping screws. Unlike the STarFix platform, which is elevated above the head on tripod-like legs, the Nexframe looks like a broad funnel with its tip attached to the skull (**Fig. 2**). The upper half of the device is dome shaped and can rotate, and a small platform on top of the dome can translate in one direction along a track. These 2 degrees of freedom allow the platform to be aimed at cranial targets that lie within an approximately 50° arc. The location of the burr hole and to some degree the curvature of the skull

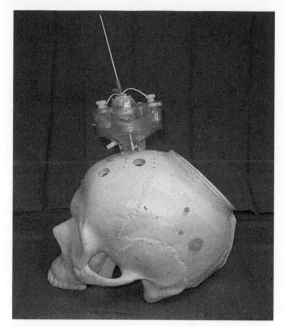

Fig. 2. The Medtronic Nexframe frameless DBS device mounted on a phantom skull.

dictates what brain regions can be targeted with the Nexframe. Although the most common targets such as the STN and thalamus can be easily reached, sometimes care must be taken with more lateral targets such as the globus pallidus. The platform contains an insert with 5 channels through which guide tubes, microelectrodes, and DBS electrodes can pass.

The bone-implanted fiducials are again placed using local anesthetic in the outpatient setting. Imaging and targeting can be performed beforehand, providing the temporal decoupling of targeting from the day of surgery that is one of the hallmarks of frameless DBS. This again allows patients to get to the operating room faster, thus minimizing their time off medications. In the operating room, registration must be performed using an infrared optical tracking system. Unlike traditional cranial applications in which the patient's head is rigidly fixed with a Mayfield-type device and the reference frame is in turn mounted to the head holder, in frameless DBS the reference frame is mounted to the Nexframe itself. The patient can therefore move his or her head during surgery if desired. The bulkiness of the Nexframe often necessitates mounting one device at a time on each side of the head for bilateral simultaneous implantations so they do not physically interfere with each other, although the author and others have experience with placing 2 Nexframes at once without incident.

TARGET LOCALIZATION

The second variable that can be readily adapted to a more minimally invasive approach is the target localization method. Both frame-based and frame-less DBS techniques use a combination of (1) some method of preoperative imaging to define the target in stereotactic space before electrode implantation, and (2) some method of physiologic confirmation that the target has been reached during electrode implantation. Methods of preoperative imaging include MRI, CT, and ventriculography. MRI has the advantage of superior tissue discrimination but is subject to image distortion due to multiple factors, including the inherent inhomogeneities in the magnetic field of all MRI scanners. CT has poor image discrimination but is free from image distortion. Many groups, therefore, use a combination of CT and MRI to perform targeting. Ventriculography was used extensively before the advent of CT and MRI, and although it is still used by some, it is itself invasive and therefore has been largely abandoned.

Methods of physiologic confirmation of target localization during surgery vary significantly based on the target being implanted, the preferences and skill set of the implanting team, the available resources, and even the surgical culture in different parts of the world. In general, the target can be localized by a combination of a micro/recording technique and a macro/stimulation technique in patients undergoing awake surgery. The most common microphysiology technique is MER, which is performed with a small-diameter, fine-tipped electrode capable of performing single-cell (or small number multiunit) neuronal recordings. MER takes advantage of the fact that areas of subcortical white matter are relatively electrically silent, whereas areas of subcortical gray matter (nuclei) are relatively active. Moreover, different nuclei have their own characteristic pattern of spontaneous neuronal activity, which are discernible to the experienced observer. In this manner, one can pass a microelectrode down through the brain to the intended target and usually determine with confidence that the proper region has been reached. Although MER is the most common method, others rely on information obtained by performing stimulation at low amplitude through a microelectrode. Some perform neuronal recordings but via a larger electrode to obtain cellular activity on a larger scale or record local field potentials. Following this micro/recording process (which is often referred to as mapping), many surgeons perform a macro/stimulation technique, often to confirm the final electrode position. Again, the actual process can vary widely, but the most common technique is to place the actual DBS electrode at the desired location and stimulate directly through it. One can observe improvement in some symptoms such as tremor and rigidity if present, and also infer the electrode position by observing adverse effects of stimulating adjacent brain structures at higher levels of stimulation.

These techniques are by definition invasive and can significantly lengthen the time of the procedure (and therefore also increase patient discomfort). In the United States, most teams perform MER with passage of a single microelectrode at a time, with the cumulative information obtained with each pass used to create a physiologic map of the intended target. Once the team feels they have obtained a sufficient amount of anatomic information, MER is stopped. Others in the United States and around the world perform MER by placing up to 5 microelectrodes in the brain and recording simultaneously from the array. The process of MER, therefore, produces somewhere between 1 and 5 brain penetrations for a typical target; this is then followed by insertion of the actual DBS electrode, which itself may be removed and repositioned based on the results of macrostimulation.

An alternative method of target localization that eliminates the need for awake, physiologic mapping with multiple brain penetrations would provide a less invasive approach to DBS surgery. Interventional MRI (iMRI) is a technique that was developed in the early and mid 1990s to allow neurosurgeons to perform cranial procedures within an MRI scanner suite. iMRI has been particularly useful for some brain tumor resections, in which MRI sequences can be obtained intraoperatively to navigate accurately, even in the face of significant brain shift during the procedure. The technique has not been adopted widely, in large part because of the extensive financial and logistical considerations of placing MRI scanners inside operating rooms. In the early 2000s, we started to consider how this method of intraoperative imaging could be applied to DBS electrode implantation. Instead of building an MRI scanner inside an existing operating room, we focused on using diagnostic scanners in the Radiology Department under sterile conditions.

1.5-T iMRI is presently used to place DBS electrodes into the STN and GPi to treat a subset of patients with PD and dystonia.[2,3] The rationale for moving in this direction was the observation that patients with PD with consistently good outcomes had leads centered in the dorsolateral STN, in line with the anterior third of the adjacent red nucleus.[4] This corresponds anatomically with the motor subterritory of the STN, the region that we seek to identify in the regular operating room through the process of MER and macrostimulation. Because the STN is visible on 1.5-T T2-weighted images, we sought to use real-time MRI to place electrodes into this location instead of using physiologic mapping. As experience with real-time MRI grew, the GPi, which is also easily visualized at 1.5 T, was targeted as well. This approach represents an evolution toward minimally invasive DBS surgery by radically altering the method of target localization. No frame or fiducials are used and no preoperative imaging is needed. As no physiologic mapping is required, the procedure can be done under general anesthesia with only one brain penetration in the overwhelming majority of cases.

iMRI-guided implantation is performed inside a 1.5-T MRI scanner (**Fig. 3**). Traditional high-grade stainless instruments cannot be used in the MR environment, so nonferrous titanium instruments and an MR-compatible pneumatic drill (Anspach, Palm Beach Gardens, FL or Stryker, Kalamazoo, MI) are used during the procedure. Instead of a stereotactic frame, a slightly modified Nexframe is used as the delivery device. This procedure is analogous to the use of the Nexframe in a regular operating room, with the important distinction that no fiducial registration and no optical tracking are required when using iMRI. In this context, the Nexframe is not used as an integrated part of a neuronavigation system, rather it becomes a passive aiming device, with the MRI scanner software acting as the interface between the anatomy and the surgeon. Unilateral or simultaneous bilateral implantations can be performed, provided the entry points are far enough apart that 2 Nexframes can be mounted without interfering with each other.

After the patient is anesthetized, the head is placed in a carbon fiber head holder to prevent inadvertent movement during the procedure. The patient is moved to the isocenter of the MRI bore, and imaging is obtained to determine the entry point and trajectory. Once the entry points are selected, the patient is moved to the distal end of the bore so that the top of the head is easily accessible. The entry points are marked on the scalp and skull using a marking pen and syringe-with methylene blue, and a custom sterile drape is used to establish an accordion-like sterile field that encompasses the distal bore and end of the magnet and allows for patient movement. Opening of the skin, burr hole creation, and mounting of the Nexframes proceeds as it would during a regular frameless case.

The patient is moved to the center of the bore for high-resolution imaging, definitive target selection,

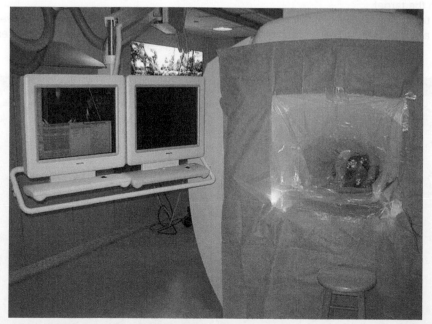

Fig. 3. Photo of a 1.5-T MRI suite during iMRI DBS. A sterile drape creates a sterile field from the distal end of the MRI machine into the bore of the scanner. The top of the patient's head is visible in the bore with bilateral Nexframe devices mounted. Monitors in the MR suite to the left allow the surgeon to see real-time images throughout the procedure.

and implantation. A saline-filled MRI visible alignment stem is placed into the Nexframe; this device has a sphere at its proximal end (actually within the burr hole) that sits at the so-called pivot point or center of rotation of the Nexframe device. The pivot point therefore remains stationary regardless of the Nexframe's orientation. The 3-dimensional coordinates for the center of the pivot point can be determined in MR space by setting up a region of interest (ROI) on its image using the MR console software. When the target is selected and its coordinates in MR space are also determined using an ROI, the target and pivot point coordinates are used to define the "target line," which represents the desired trajectory to the target. The surgeon can reach in to the bore of the magnet and move the Nexframe until the alignment stem is aligned with the target line. A rapid MR acquisition at a rate of 3 to 5 images per second allows the surgeon to visualize the fluid stem during this process in real time. The Nexframe is locked into position, proper alignment is ensured by obtaining additional images, and if no further adjustments are needed a ceramic stylet inside a peel-away sheath is inserted and advanced to the target (**Fig. 4**). Once proper placement is confirmed with high-resolution MRI, the stylet is removed and the DBS lead is placed down the peel-away sheath to the target. High-resolution images are used to confirm final lead position and the peel-away heath is subsequently removed, leaving the DBS lead in the target.

The iMRI technique has several advantages that qualify it as a minimally invasive approach for DBS implantation. It does not require fiducial or frame placement and does not require any preoperative imaging. Moreover, there is no intraoperative physiology necessary, which results in significant time saved over traditional implantation techniques. The patients do not have to be awake or be off medications, which greatly increases patient comfort. The implantation can be done with one penetration of the brain as opposed to multiple penetrations used in physiologically mapped cases, which may eventually be shown to decrease the risk of hemorrhage. Finally, there is a high degree of confidence that the lead is placed in a favorable position prior to the end of the procedure. One disadvantage is that at present, the procedure requires a significant amount of technical expertise from an MR physicist to run the MR scanner. The Nexframe and MR console software are not designed optimally to perform this type of intervention, and possess inherent deficiencies that can create technical challenges during the procedure. A new hardware and software system has been developed specifically for iMRI procedures that addresses many of these shortcomings.[5,6] iMRI also requires institutional commitment to using MRI scanners for interventional procedures and radiology, anesthesia, and operating room personnel who are willing to work in this unique environment.

MODULATION HARDWARE

A final way to make surgery for movement disorders more minimally invasive is to eliminate the

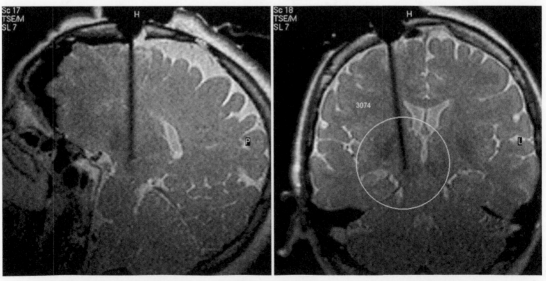

Fig. 4. Intraoperative MR images during an iMRI DBS case. Images obtained at 90° to each other in plane with the target trajectory show a ceramic stylet and peel-away sheath that has been placed in the right STN.

implanted hardware completely and modulate the structures of interest biologically. Although DBS is an effective treatment for movement disorders, it is a hardware-based therapy and is therefore subject to the complexities and potential complications of implanting foreign objects into the body. Lead migration or fracture, skin erosion, and pulse generator failure are all complications that are unique to DBS, and published infection rates in DBS are higher than those seen with other stereotactic procedures that do not involve implanted hardware.[7] In addition, DBS is a time-intensive therapy after surgery, with multiple office visits required to optimize stimulator settings and to balance the effects of stimulation and medication. Finally, DBS is a battery-driven device and requires periodic surgical replacement of the pulse generator that powers the system.

Because PD in particular is caused by degeneration of a well-characterized population of neurons, investigators have long sought a surgical therapy that would "replace" the lost biologic function in this disorder. Although various cell transplantation trials have been disappointing to date, there is presently a strong interest in gene transfer as a potential treatment for PD. Gene transfer uses a viral vector to carry a gene interest into neurons in a particular brain target. The transduced neurons then produce a new protein product; in the gene therapy trials that have been done so far, this product has been either an enzyme that alters local biology or a growth factor that supports and protects local or even distant cells.[8–10] The viral vector for all of these trials has been adeno-associated virus that is selected for a variety of reasons including its lack of pathogenicity, its minimal immune response, and its ability to predictably integrate into the genome of nondividing cells in a stable manner.

From a surgical standpoint, gene transfer for PD so far has been performed using traditional frame-based stereotaxy (**Fig. 5**). The procedures have varied depending on the target of interest. One study involved gene transfer to the STN and used MER for target localization, as the physiologic characteristics of that nucleus are well understood.[9] Other studies targeted the putamen, and as this is not a target well characterized physiologically, the procedures were done strictly on an anatomic basis. The number of cannulas passed to the target regions varied as well, with up to 4 penetrations per putamen being performed in one trial.[10] Delivery of vector was achieved by either intermittent hand injection or pump-driven convection enhanced delivery.

Although these procedures do not meet criteria for minimally invasive surgery based on the

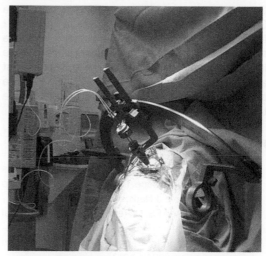

Fig. 5. Intraoperative photo during a gene transfer case for Parkinson disease. A standard stereotactic frame is being used, with infusion occurring through 2 custom-designed cannulas placed in the putamen.

number of brain penetrations, a unique delivery device, or target localization method, they deserve mention because they do not involve any implanted hardware at all. These procedures therefore avoid all of the potential complications associated with a hardware-based therapy, and are generally thought to have a lower infection rate than DBS. Gene transfer is also in theory a low-maintenance therapy for patients, because they do not require device programming or battery replacements. Future gene transfer trials that will reduce the number of cannula penetrations required are in the planning stages, and use iMRI for targeting as well as real-time visualization of the infusions; animal studies using these techniques are currently under way.[11]

SUMMARY

Although surgery for movement disorders is already a minimally invasive endeavor, the pursuit of less invasive surgery is a noble one regardless of the subspecialty. New frameless stereotactic delivery devices, novel ways of localizing brain targets using real-time imaging, and biologic strategies such as gene transfer are paving the way to shorter, safer, and less traumatic procedures for movement disorders patients.

ACKNOWLEDGMENTS

The author would like to thank Dr Philip Starr, Dr Alastair Martin, and Dr Jill Ostrem who are coinvestigators in the iMRI program. The author would like to thank Monica Volz, Robin Taylor, and Jamie Grace who provided nursing and research support for some of the work described in this article. The author would also like to thank and acknowledge IGN, Medtronic, and Surgivision for their past and present support of iMRI DBS, and Ceregene and Genzyme for their ongoing support of gene transfer for PD.

REFERENCES

1. Holloway KL, Gaede SE, Starr PA, et al. Frameless stereotaxy using bone fiducial markers for deep brain stimulation. J Neurosurg 2005;103:404.

2. Martin AJ, Larson PS, Ostrem JL, et al. Interventional magnetic resonance guidance of deep brain stimulator implantation for Parkinson disease. Top Magn Reson Imaging 2009;19:213.

3. Starr PA, Martin AJ, Ostrem JL, et al. Subthalamic nucleus deep brain stimulator placement using high-field interventional magnetic resonance imaging and a skull-mounted aiming device: technique and application accuracy. J Neurosurg 2010; 112(3):479–90.

4. Starr PA, Christine CW, Theodosopoulos PV, et al. Implantation of deep brain stimulators into the sub-thalamic nucleus: technical approach and magnetic resonance imaging-verified lead locations. J Neurosurg 2002;97:370.

5. Barbre CJ. Devices for targeting the needle. Neurosurg Clin N Am 2009;20:187.

6. Martin AJ, Starr PA, Larson PS. Software requirements for interventional MR in restorative and functional neurosurgery. Neurosurg Clin N Am 2009;20:179.

7. Sillay KA, Larson PS, Starr PA. Deep brain stimulator hardware-related infections: incidence and management in a large series. Neurosurgery 2008;62:360.

8. Christine CW, Starr PA, Larson PS, et al. Safety and tolerability of putaminal AADC gene therapy for Parkinson disease. Neurology 2009;73:1662.

9. Kaplitt MG, Feigin A, Tang C, et al. Safety and tolerability of gene therapy with an adeno-associated virus (AAV) borne GAD gene for Parkinson's disease: an open label, phase I trial. Lancet 2007; 369:2097.

10. Marks WJ Jr, Ostrem JL, Verhagen L, et al. Safety and tolerability of intraputaminal delivery of CERE-120 (adeno-associated virus serotype 2-neurturin) to patients with idiopathic Parkinson's disease: an open-label, phase I trial. Lancet Neurol 2008;7:400.

11. Gimenez F, Krauze MT, Valles F, et al. Image-guided convection-enhanced delivery of GDNF protein into monkey putamen. Neuroimage 2010. [Epub ahead of print].

Complication Avoidance in Minimally Invasive Neurosurgery

Michael E. Sughrue, MD[a],*, Steven A. Mills, BFA[a],
Ronald L. Young II, MD[b]

KEYWORDS

- Complication • Endoscopic • Outcome • Avoidance

Although minimally invasive neurosurgery (MIN) holds the potential for reducing the approach-related impact on normal brain, bone, and soft tissues, which must be manipulated in more conventional transcranial microneurosurgery, the techniques necessary to perform minimally invasive, yet maximally effective neurosurgery place significant demands on the surgeon because in many ways the more limited exposure creates a number of unique ways these operations can go wrong. Safe and effective MIN requires the conscious institution of specific alterations to the surgeon's usual operative case flow, which are designed to make specific well-known mistakes impossible or at least very unlikely. Thus, it is important for the aspiring MIN surgeons to learn from the mistakes of their predecessors and to institute patterns of behavior that prevent a repetition of these mistakes. This article provides practical information regarding known pitfalls in intraventricular and transcranial neuroendoscopic surgeries and provides practical methods to reduce the incidence of these complications to the lowest rate possible.

PITFALL #1: LACK OF NECESSARY EQUIPMENT OR EQUIPMENT FAILURE

This pitfall category roughly encompasses a large number of potential mistakes, all of which are significantly problematic and avoidable. It is important to view endoscopic surgery in the model of the airline industry, in that the beginning of each procedure should involve a systematic and stereotyped evaluation of the equipment needed to perform the procedure in question. Most importantly, the presence of each endoscope needed to perform the planned procedure needs to be confirmed, and the function and image quality of these endoscopes need to be evaluated. Ideally, this evaluation should be performed before the induction of general anesthesia but certainly must be done before skin incision. Further, all working cannulas or sheaths and all introducing devices need to be present and confirmed to be correct for the endoscopes in use. If specifically instrumentation (eg, monopolar cautery, graspers, suction tubing) is needed, it should be confirmed that it is present and functioning and that it will fit down the working channel of the endoscope used. If image guidance is to be used, it should be confirmed to be appropriately registered and to have image probes or other device adapters appropriate for the planned case.

In addition, it is important that the instrumentation is confirmed to be setup and working appropriately before skin incision. The foramen of Monro is not the correct time and place to troubleshoot problems with the monitors, incorrect up-down orientation with the endoscope, and malfunctioning irrigation channels. A systematic checklist approach is the key to avoid these frustrating errors.

[a] Department of Neurological Surgery, University of California at San Francisco, 505 Parnassus Avenue, San Francisco, CA 94117, USA
[b] Indianapolis Neurosurgery, 8333 Naab Road, Suite 250, Indianapolis, IN 46260, USA
* Corresponding author.
E-mail address: SughrueM@Neurosurg.UCSF.Edu

Neurosurg Clin N Am 21 (2010) 699–702
doi:10.1016/j.nec.2010.07.006
1042-3680/10/$ — see front matter © 2010 Elsevier Inc. All rights reserved.

PITFALL #2: INAPPROPRIATE PREOPERATIVE PLANNING

Given the keyhole emphasis of MIN, MIN exposures tend to expose less and are thus less flexible than larger exposures. Openings are targeted to the pathology in question and are not robust to large inappropriate deviations from the ideal trajectory. Hence, it is important to spend more time with this approach than one would spend with a larger approach, considering the implications of specific aspects of the intended trajectory. Although some procedures (notably third ventriculostomy) can be performed using stereotyped entry points, most procedures require a thoughtful case-by-case assessment of the individual lesion being treated and its relationship to critical normal structures. Although planning these cases becomes more intuitive with experience, image guidance can be invaluable to those less experienced with MIN. For complicated intraventricular or intracranial lesions, the use of image guidance to plan an idea trajectory and to adhere to this plan is indispensible, and an excellent image registration should be viewed as a critical part of technical success.

PITFALL #3: GETTING LOST

Second only to beginning the procedure without the appropriate equipment, getting lost is the greatest sin of minimally invasive intraventricular or intracranial surgery, and without conscious efforts to avoid getting lost, it is an easier state to achieve than one would initially think is possible. An inaccurate or inappropriate understanding of the anatomy visualized can provide the unwary surgeon with a false sense of what areas are safe and what areas to avoid, prompting inappropriate actions, with potentially devastating results. A thorough familiarity with the anatomy obtained through dissections and experience obviously lowers the risk of getting lost, especially when combined with image guidance.

There are several common regions encountered during ventriculoscopy that even those familiar with the relevant anatomy can misinterpret, if not aware of these possible mistakes. One well-known error is unknowingly entering the contralateral lateral ventricle, which if not recognized can cause the surgeon to inappropriately enter the wrong foramen of Monro, causing traction and potential injury to both fornices. Another error is mistaking the cerebral aqueduct for the infundibular recess of the third ventricle. Such a misinterpretation can cause the surgeon to perform a third ventriculostomy, just posterior to the mamillary bodies (which is interpreted as being anterior to the mamillary bodies), with devastating injury to the midbrain and/or basilar artery. Hence, it is critical that after gaining ventricular access with the endoscope the surgeon survey the anatomy carefully before making any definitive maneuvers. The choice of correct trajectory, the appropriate confirmation and maintenance of a correct up-down orientation of the endoscope, and the use of image guidance are also important for avoiding these kinds of mistakes. However, the importance of a slow and deliberate assessment of the orientation provided is essential to avoid getting lost.

PITFALL #4: INAPPROPRIATE POSITIONING

Appropriate patient positioning for MIN goes hand in hand with preoperative planning. Although some procedures can be performed using stereotyped room arrangements and patient positioning, it is important to consciously assess the effect of the planned position in the context of the planned trajectory. If the planned position makes the ideal trajectory awkward, then the risk of deviating from this trajectory is higher, thus increasing the possibility of obtaining problematic or disorienting anatomic views as described earlier.

Further, for transcranial endoscope-assisted procedures, good patient positioning can maximize gravity brain retraction and obviate the need for physical brain retractors, which is doubtlessly better for the patient.

PITFALL #5: FAILED ATTEMPTS TO ACCESS THE VENTRICLE

Most endoscopes used in intraventricular endoscopy are much larger than ventricular catheters that neurosurgeons use for cerebrospinal fluid diversion procedures. It is hypothesized that larger diameter instruments cause greater tearing of white matter tracts than ventricular catheters. This feature makes inappropriate passes into the thalamus, internal capsule, brainstem, and basal ganglia a potential devastating complication of misguided attempts to enter the ventricle with the endoscope. Although good preoperative planning and the use of image guidance can reduce this risk, they cannot eliminate it because some brain shift is inevitable upon dural entry. It is critical to first tap the ventricle with a smaller gauge cannula or ventricular catheter to ensure that the planned trajectory is into the ventricle and that the anatomy is roughly as anticipated.

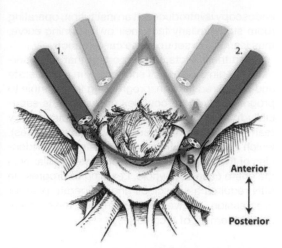

Fig. 1. A comparison of methods for redirecting the position of the endoscope from position 1 to position 2. The trajectories for the incorrect (B) slashing maneuver and correct (A) fencing maneuver for lateral movement of the endoscope are compared to highlight the potential consequences of the slashing maneuver in an anatomically critical position.

PITFALL #6: INAPPROPRIATE MOVEMENT OF THE ENDOSCOPE

Learning to avoid this complication requires a conscious effort to alter one's instinct to decide that a nearby structure in the peripheral portion of the field of endoscopic vision is of interest and to swing the endoscope laterally to visualize this structure. The risk of such maneuvers is indicated in **Fig. 1**. As demonstrated, these lateral sweeping maneuvers risk injuring or tearing all structures within the angle subtended by this sweeping motion. MIN surgeons need to consciously train themselves to maneuver the endoscope laterally using a fencing motion as opposed to a slashing motion (see **Fig. 1**), which is best perfected with practical exercises on cadavers.

PITFALL #7: FAILURE TO APPRECIATE THE ENDOSCOPE'S BLIND SPOT

One principle advantage of the endoscope is its ability to place the light and view sources as close to the area of interest as possible, thus limiting interference from more proximal overlying structures. One of its most dangerous features is that when the endoscope is placed close to the region of interest, the surgeon's ability to appropriately visualize much of the pathway between the skin and the target becomes minimal (**Fig. 2**A). This trait creates the potential for instruments to unknowingly injure important structures on the way in, if blindly introduced. MIN surgeons must consciously train themselves to remove the endoscope with the insertion of each new instrument and to follow the instrument into the field under direct endoscopic visualization.

A corollary of the endoscopic blind spot is the potential for the endoscope to inadvertently strike or cause pressure injury to unseen structures behind it (see **Fig. 2**B). This potential is most important during transcranial endoscopic surgery because endoscopic visualization of deeper intracranial structures can place critical structures, such as the optic nerve, in the blind spot where it can be injured by the endoscope that is out of view. This injury can be avoided by continuous visual monitoring of the endoscope shaft's location by the surgical assistant who observes the endoscope through the microscope and prevents contact with important structures, such as the optic nerve.

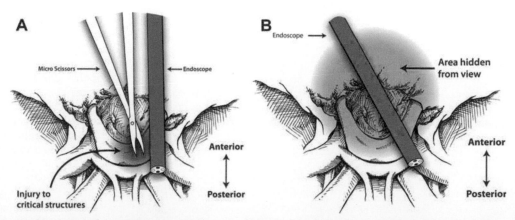

Fig. 2. The blind spot of the endoscope. (*A*) The risk of blindly introducing instruments without direct endoscopic visualization. (*B*) The risk of not being aware of the position of the endoscope shaft.

PITFALL #8: BITING OFF MORE THAN YOU CAN CHEW

Like microsurgery, endoscopic neurosurgery is a skill set which improves with use, and there is a learning curve. The views are often unfamiliar, and disorientation is easier than with the microscope, especially during the transition from the microscope to the endoscope. The methods for dealing with problems such as bleeding in an endoscopic approach are different from those in microsurgery, and many neurosurgeons feel less in control at first. Further, many good habits such as using correct techniques for moving the endoscope and introducing instruments must be consciously adopted and reinforced through practice. As

endoscopy is introduced at an institution, operating room staff similarly face their own learning curve, thus learning to set up these cases effectively.

Given these facts, it is important that neurosurgeons begin their use of endoscopy in a deliberate and measured fashion, progressing from simple to progressively more complex cases. This is especially true with cases involving a multidisciplinary team-based approach (such as endonasal cases), which add the additional need to learn the tendencies of the cosurgeon and to become familiar with the entire case as a whole. Learning to progress in MIN requires a conscious and deliberate plan for progression, as well as continuous assessment and refinement of techniques.

Index

Neurosurg Clin N Am 21 (2010) 703–707
doi:10.1016/S1042-3680(10)00087-2
1042-3680/10/$ – see front matter © 2010 Elsevier Inc. All rights reserved

United States Postal Service

Statement of Ownership, Management, and Circulation
(All Periodicals Publications Except Requestor Publications)

1. Publication Title	2. Publication Number	3. Filing Date
Neurosurgery Clinics of North America	0 1 3 - 1 2 4	9/15/10

4. Issue Frequency	5. Number of Issues Published Annually	6. Annual Subscription Price
Jan, Apr, Jul, Oct	4	$296.00

7. Complete Mailing Address of Known Office of Publication (Not printer) (Street, city, county, state, and ZIP+4®)

Elsevier Inc.
360 Park Avenue South
New York, NY 10010-1710

Contact Person: Stephen Bushing
Telephone (Include area code): 215-239-3688

8. Complete Mailing Address of Headquarters or General Business Office of Publisher (Not printer)

Elsevier Inc., 360 Park Avenue South, New York, NY 10010-1710

9. Full Names and Complete Mailing Addresses of Publisher, Editor, and Managing Editor (Do not leave blank)

Publisher (Name and complete mailing address)

Kim Murphy, Elsevier, Inc., 1600 John F. Kennedy Blvd. Suite 1800, Philadelphia, PA 19103-2899

Editor (Name and complete mailing address)

Ruth Malwitz, Elsevier, Inc., 1600 John F. Kennedy Blvd. Suite 1800, Philadelphia, PA 19103-2899

Managing Editor (Name and complete mailing address)

Catherine Bewick, Elsevier, Inc., 1600 John F. Kennedy Blvd. Suite 1800, Philadelphia, PA 19103-2899

10. Owner (Do not leave blank. If the publication is owned by a corporation, give the name and address of the corporation immediately followed by the names and addresses of all stockholders owning or holding 1 percent or more of the total amount of stock. If not owned by a corporation, give the names and addresses of the individual owners. If owned by a partnership or other unincorporated firm, give its name and address as well as those of each individual owner. If the publication is published by a nonprofit organization, give its name and address.)

Full Name	Complete Mailing Address
Wholly owned subsidiary of	4520 East-West Highway
Reed/Elsevier, US holdings	Bethesda, MD 20814

11. Known Bondholders, Mortgagees, and Other Security Holders Owning or Holding 1 Percent or More of Total Amount of Bonds, Mortgages, or Other Securities. If none, check box ☐ None

Full Name	Complete Mailing Address
N/A	

12. Tax Status (For completion by nonprofit organizations authorized to mail at nonprofit rates) (Check one)
The purpose, function, and nonprofit status of this organization and the exempt status for federal income tax purposes:
☐ Has Not Changed During Preceding 12 Months
☐ Has Changed During Preceding 12 Months (Publisher must submit explanation of change with this statement)

PS Form 3526, September 2007 (Page 1 of 3 Instructions Page 3)) PSN 7530-01-000-9931 PRIVACY NOTICE: See our Privacy policy in www.usps.com

---

13. Publication Title	14. Issue Date for Circulation Data Below
Neurosurgery Clinics of North America	July 2010

15. Extent and Nature of Circulation		Average No. Copies Each Issue During Preceding 12 Months	No. Copies of Single Issue Published Nearest to Filing Date
a. Total Number of Copies (Net press run)		1176	1100
b. Paid Circulation (By Mail and Outside the Mail)	(1) Mailed Outside-County Paid Subscriptions Stated on PS Form 3541. (Include paid distribution above nominal rate, advertiser's proof copies, and exchange copies)	387	376
	(2) Mailed In-County Paid Subscriptions Stated on PS Form 3541 (Include paid distribution above nominal rate, advertiser's proof copies, and exchange copies)		
	(3) Paid Distribution Outside the Mails Including Sales Through Dealers and Carriers, Street Vendors, Counter Sales, and Other Paid Distribution Outside USPS®	214	213
	(4) Paid Distribution by Other Classes Mailed Through the USPS (e.g. First-Class Mail®)		
c. Total Paid Distribution (Sum of 15b (1), (2), (3), and (4))	►	601	589
d. Free or Nominal Rate Distribution (By Mail and Outside the Mail)	(1) Free or Nominal Rate Outside-County Copies Included on PS Form 3541	57	55
	(2) Free or Nominal Rate In-County Copies Included on PS Form 3541		
	(3) Free or Nominal Rate Copies Mailed at Other Classes Through the USPS (e.g. First-Class Mail)		
	(4) Free or Nominal Rate Distribution Outside the Mail (Carriers or other means)		
e. Total Free or Nominal Rate Distribution (Sum of 15d (1), (2), (3) and (4))	►	57	55
f. Total Distribution (Sum of 15c and 15e)	►	658	644
g. Copies not Distributed (See instructions to publishers #4 (page #3))	►	518	456
h. Total (Sum of 15f and g)	►	1176	1100
i. Percent Paid (15c divided by 15f times 100)	►	91.34%	91.46%

16. Publication of Statement of Ownership
☐ If the publication is a general publication, publication of this statement is required. Will be printed in the October 2010 issue of this publication.   ☐ Publication not required

17. Signature and Title of Editor, Publisher, Business Manager, or Owner

Stephen R. Bushing

Stephen R. Bushing – Fulfillment/Inventory Specialist

Date: September 15, 2010

I certify that all information furnished on this form is true and complete. I understand that anyone who furnishes false or misleading information on this form or who omits material or information requested on the form may be subject to criminal sanctions (including fines and imprisonment) and/or civil sanctions (including civil penalties)

PS Form 3526, September 2007 (Page 2 of 3)

Moving?

Make sure your subscription moves with you!

To notify us of your new address, find your **Clinics Account Number** (located on your mailing label above your name), and contact customer service at:

Email: journalscustomerservice-usa@elsevier.com

800-654-2452 (subscribers in the U.S. & Canada)
314-447-8871 (subscribers outside of the U.S. & Canada)

Fax number: 314-447-8029

Elsevier Health Sciences Division
Subscription Customer Service
3251 Riverport Lane
Maryland Heights, MO 63043

*To ensure uninterrupted delivery of your subscription, please notify us at least 4 weeks in advance of move.

Printed and bound by CPI Group (UK) Ltd, Croydon, CR0 4YY

03/10/2024

01040358-0004